AMOR AND PSYCHE

THE PSYCHIC DEVELOPMENT

OF THE FEMININE

A COMMENTARY ON THE TALE BY APULEIUS

AMOR
AND PSYCHE

THE PSYCHIC DEVELOPMENT

OF THE FEMININE

A COMMENTARY ON THE TALE BY APULEIUS

BY ERICH NEUMANN

TRANSLATED FROM THE GERMAN BY

RALPH MANHEIM

HARPER TORCHBOOKS / THE BOLLINGEN LIBRARY

HARPER & ROW, PUBLISHERS

NEW YORK AND EVANSTON

AMOR AND PSYCHE

Copyright © 1956 by Bollingen Foundation Inc., New York, N.Y.

Printed in the United States of America

THIS VOLUME IS THE FIFTY-FOURTH IN A SERIES OF BOOKS
PUBLISHED BY BOLLINGEN FOUNDATION

This book was originally published in German as *Apuleius: Amor und
Psyche, mit einem Kommentar von Erich Neumann: Ein Beitrag zur
seelischen Entwicklung des Weiblichen* by Rascher Verlag, Zurich, 1952.
It was first published in English in 1956 by Pantheon Books, Inc.,
New York, for Bollingen Foundation, and is reprinted by arrangement.

First HARPER TORCHBOOK edition published 1962 by
Harper & Row, Publishers, Incorporated
New York and Evanston

Library of Congress catalog card number: 56-10425

CONTENTS

EDITORIAL NOTE

The text used for the tale of Amor and Psyche is from H. E. Butler's translation of *The Metamorphoses or Golden Ass of Apuleius of Madaura*, published at the Clarendon Press, Oxford, 1910, in two volumes, and used with the permission of the Press. Archaic forms of address have been changed to modern forms except in passages where a mortal addresses a god or goddess, or a creature or inanimate thing addresses a mortal. In a few other cases, the language has been modified to remove rather extreme archaisms or to conform with the German translation (by Albrecht Schaeffer) originally used by Dr. Neumann, where this was necessary to bring out Dr. Neumann's meaning. In general, the name of the god is given as Amor throughout the tale rather than Cupid.

Acknowledgment is gratefully made, also, to the Hogarth Press for a quotation from J. B. Leishman's translation of Rainer Maria Rilke's *Poems*; to Farrar, Straus, and Cudahy for a passage from Robert Graves' translation of *The Golden Ass* (U.S. copyright 1951 by Robert Graves); and to Miss Emily Chisholm for a passage from her unpublished translation of Rilke's "Alcestis."

THE TALE

Amor and Psyche
from the METAMORPHOSES *or* GOLDEN ASS
of Lucius *Apuleius*

BASED ON THE TRANSLATION OF H. E. BUTLER

AMOR AND PSYCHE

I**N** a certain city there once lived a king and queen. They had three daughters very fair to view. But whereas it was thought that the charms of the two eldest, great as they were, could yet be worthily celebrated by mortal praise, the youngest daughter was so strangely and wonderfully fair that human speech was all too poor to describe her beauty, or even to tell of its praise. Many of the citizens and multitudes of strangers were drawn to the town in eager crowds by the fame of so marvelous a sight and were struck dumb at the sight of such unapproachable loveliness, so that, raising their right hands to their lips, with thumb erect and the first finger laid to its base, they worshiped her with prayers of adoration as though she were the goddess Venus herself. And now the fame had gone abroad, through all the neighboring towns and all the country round about, that the goddess, who sprang from the blue deep of the sea and was born from the spray of the foaming waves, had deigned to manifest her godhead to all the world and was dwelling among earthly folk; or, if that was not so, it was certain, they said, that heaven had rained fresh procreative dew, and earth, not sea, had brought forth as a flower a second Venus in all the glory of her maidenhood.

This new belief increased each day, until it knew no bounds. The fame thereof had already spread abroad to the nearest islands and had traversed many a province and a great portion of the earth. And now many a mortal journeyed from far and sailed over the great deeps of ocean, flocking to see the wonder and glory of the age. Now no man sailed to Paphos or Cnidos, or even to Cythera, that they might behold the goddess Venus; her rites were put aside, her temples fell to ruin, her sacred couches were disregarded, her ceremonies neglected, her images uncrowned, her altars desolate and foul with fireless ashes. It was to a girl men prayed, and it was in the worship of mortal beauty that they sought to appease the power of the great goddess. When the maid went forth at morning, men propitiated the name of Venus with feast and sacrifice, though Venus was not there; and as the maid moved through the streets, multitudes prayed to her and offered flowers woven in garlands or scattered loose at will.

But the true Venus was exceedingly angry that divine honors should be transferred thus extravagantly to the worship of a mortal maid. She could bear her fury no longer, her head shook, a deep groan burst from her lips, and thus she spoke with herself: "Behold, I the first parent of created things, the primal source of all the elements; behold, I Venus, the kindly mother of all the world, must share my majesty and honor with a mortal maid, and my name that dwells in the heavens is dragged through the earthly muck. Shall I endure the doubt cast by this vicarious adoration, this worship of my godhead that is shared with her? Shall a girl that is doomed to die parade in my likeness? It was in vain the shepherd, on whose impartial justice Jove set the seal of his approval, preferred me over such mighty goddesses for my surpassing beauty. But this girl, whoever she be, that has usurped my honors shall have no joy thereof. I will make her repent of her beauty, even her unlawful loveliness."

Straightway she summoned her winged headstrong boy, that wicked boy, scorner of law and order, who, armed with arrows and torch aflame, speeds through others' homes by night, saps the ties of wedlock, and all unpunished commits hideous crime and uses all his power for ill. Him then, though wantonness and lust are his by birth, she fired still further by her words, and leading him to that city showed him Psyche—for so the maid was called—face to face. Then, groaning at the far-flown renown of her fair rival, her utterance broken with indignation, she cried: "I implore you by all the bonds of love that bind you to her that bore you, by the sweet wounds your arrows deal and by the honeyed smart of your fires, avenge your mother, yes, avenge her to the full and sternly punish this rebellious beauty. But this, this only, this beyond all else I would have you do and do with a will. Cause the maid to be consumed with passion for the vilest of men, for one whom Fortune has condemned to have neither health, nor wealth, nor honor, one so broken that through all the world his misery has no peer."

So spoke she, and with parted lips kissed her son long and fervently. Then she returned to the shore hard by, where the sea ebbs and flows, and treading with rosy feet the topmost foam of the quivering waves, plunged down to the deep's dry floor. The sea gods tarried not to do her service. It was as though she had long since commanded their presence, though in truth she had but just formed the wish. The daughters of Nereus came singing in harmony, Neptune, also called Portunus, came with bristling beard of azure, his wife Salacia with fish-teeming womb, and their babe Palaemon, rider of the dolphin. Now far and wide hosts of Tritons came plunging through the seas; one blew a soft blast from his echoing shell, another with a silken awning shaded her head from the fierce heat of the sun, a third held up a mirror before his mistress's eyes, while others swam yoked beneath her car. Such was the host that escorted Venus, as she went on her way to the halls of ocean.

Meanwhile Psyche, for all her manifest beauty, had no joy of her loveliness. All men gazed upon her, yet never a king nor prince nor even a lover from the common folk came forward desirous to claim her hand in marriage. Men marveled at her divine loveliness, but as men marvel at a statue fairly wrought. Long since, her elder sisters, whose beauty was but ordinary and had never been praised through all the world, had been betrothed to kings who came to woo, and they had become happy brides. But Psyche sat at home an unwedded maid and, sick of body and broken in spirit, bewailed her loneliness and solitude, loathing in her heart the loveliness that had charmed so many nations. Wherefore the father of the hapless girl was seized with great grief; suspecting the anger of heaven and fearing the wrath of the gods, he inquired of the most ancient oracle of the Milesian god, and with prayer and burnt offering besought the mighty deity to send a husband to wed the maid whom none had wooed.

Apollo, though an Ionian and a Greek, in order not to

embarrass the author of this Milesian tale delivered his
oracle in Latin as follows:

On some high crag, O king, set forth the maid,
In all the pomp of funeral robes arrayed.
Hope for no bridegroom born of mortal seed,
But fierce and wild and of the dragon breed.
He swoops all-conquering, borne on airy wing,
With fire and sword he makes his harvesting;
Trembles before him Jove, whom gods do dread,
And quakes the darksome river of the dead.

The king, once so happy, on hearing the pronouncement
of the sacred oracle returned home in sorrow and distress
and set forth to his wife the things ordained in that ill-
starred oracle. They mourned and wept and lamented for
many days. But at last the time drew near for the loathsome
performance of that cruel ordinance. The unhappy maid
was arrayed for her ghastly bridal, the torches' flame
burned low, clogged with dark soot and ash, the strains
of the flute of wedlock were changed to the melancholy
Lydian mode, the glad chant of the hymeneal hymn
ended in mournful wailing, and the girl on the eve of
marriage wiped away her tears even with her bridal
veil. The whole city also joined in weeping the sad fate
of the stricken house, and the public grief found expression in an edict suspending all business.

But the commands of heaven must be obeyed, and the
unhappy Psyche must go to meet her doom. And so
when all the rites of this ghastly bridal had been performed amid deepest grief, the funeral train of the
living dead was led forth escorted by all the people. It

was not her marriage procession that Psyche followed dissolved in tears, but her own obsequies. Bowed in grief and overwhelmed by their sore calamity, her parents still shrank to perform the hateful deed. But their daughter herself addressed them thus:

"Why torment your hapless age with this long weeping? Why with ceaseless wailing weary the life within you, life more near and dear to me than to yourselves? Why with vain tears deform those features that I so revere? Why lacerate your eyes? Your eyes are mine! Why beat your bosoms and the breasts that suckled me? Lo! what rich recompense you have for my glorious beauty! Too late you perceive that the mortal blow that strikes you down is dealt by wicked Envy. When nations and peoples gave me divine honor, when with one voice they hailed me as a new Venus, then was the time for you to grieve, to weep and mourn me as one dead. Now I perceive, now my eyes are opened. It is the name of Venus and that alone which has brought me to my death. Lead me on and set me on the crag that fate has appointed. I hasten to meet that blest union, I hasten to behold the noble husband that awaits me. Why do I put off and shun his coming? Was he not born to destroy all the world?"

So spoke the maid and then was silent, and with step unwavering mingled in the crowd of folk that followed to do her honor. They climbed a lofty mountain and came to the appointed crag. There they placed the maiden on the topmost peak and all departed from her. The marriage torches, with which they had lit the way before her, were all extinguished by their tears. They left them and with downcast heads prepared to return home. As for her hapless parents, crushed by the weight of their calamity, they shut themselves within their house of gloom and gave themselves over to perpetual night. Psyche meanwhile sat trembling and afraid upon the very summit of the crag and wept, when suddenly a soft air from the breathing West made her raiment wave and blew out the tunic of her bosom, then gradually raised her and, bearing her slowly on its quiet breath down the slopes of that high cliff, let her fall gently down and laid her on the flowery sward in the bosom of a deep vale.

Psyche lay sweetly reclined in that soft grassy place on a couch of herbage fresh with dew. Her wild anguish of spirit was assuaged and she fell softly asleep. When she had slumbered enough and was refreshed, she rose to her feet. The tempest had passed from her soul. She beheld a grove of huge and lofty trees, she beheld a transparent fountain of glassy water. In the very heart of the grove beside the gliding stream there stood a palace, built by no human hands but by the cunning of a god. You will perceive, as soon as I have taken you within, that it is the pleasant and luxurious dwelling of some deity that I present to your gaze. For the fretted roof on high was curiously carved of sandalwood and ivory, and the columns that upheld it were of gold. All the walls were covered with wild beasts and creatures of the field, wrought in chased silver, and confronting the gaze of those who entered. Truly it must be some demigod, or rather in very truth a god, that had power by the subtlety of his matchless skill to put such wild life into silver. The pavement was of precious stones cut small and patterned with images of many kinds. Most surely, yes, again and yet again I say it, blessed are those whose feet tread upon gems and jewels. The rest of the house through all its length and breadth was precious beyond price. All the walls were built of solid ingots of gold and shone with peculiar splendor, making a daylight of their own within the house, even though the sun should withhold his beams. Such were the lightnings flashed from bedchamber and colonnade and from the very doors themselves. Nor were the riches in the rest of the house unworthy of such splendor. It seemed a heavenly palace built by great Jove that he might dwell with mortal men.

Allured by the charm and beauty of the place, Psyche drew near and, as her confidence increased, crossed the threshold. Soon the delight of gazing on such loveliness drew her on to explore each glory, until at last on the farther side of the house she beheld a lofty chamber piled high with countless treasure. Nothing may be found in all the world that was not there. But wondrous as was the sight of such vast wealth, yet more marvelous was it that there was no chain nor bar nor sentinel to guard the treasure of all the world. Deep joy filled her at the sight, when suddenly a bodiless voice spoke to her: "Why, lady," it said, "are you overwhelmed at the sight of so great wealth? All is yours. Go now to your chamber, refresh your weariness upon your couch, and bathe when it pleases you so to do. We whose voices you hear are your servants who will wait upon you diligently and, when you have refreshed your body, will straightway serve you with a royal banquet."

When she heard these disembodied voices Psyche perceived that their instructions and all the treasure of the palace must be the gift of some god that watched over her. First for a while she slept, then, waking, bathed to refresh her weariness. This done, she beheld hard by a couch shaped like a half-moon, and, deeming from the dinner service spread beside it that it was meant for her refreshment, gladly lay down. Forthwith she was served with wine like nectar and many a delicious dish. Still no one waited on her, but all things seemed wafted to her as it were by some wind. Neither could she see any person, she only heard words that fell from the air, and none save voices were her servants. After she had feasted thus daintily, one whom she could not see entered and sang to her, while another struck the lyre, though never a lyre was to be seen. Then the harmony of a multitude of musicians was borne to her ears, so that she knew that a choir was there, though no one was visible. These delights over, Psyche went to her bed, for the hour was late.

Now when night was well advanced a soft sound came to her ears. She trembled for her honor, seeing that she was all alone; she shook for terror, and her fear of the unknown surpassed by far the fear of any peril that ever she had conceived. At length her unknown husband came and climbed the couch, made Psyche his bride, and departed in haste before the dawn. And forthwith the voices came to her chamber and served all her needs. So for a long time her life passed by, till at length, as nature ordains, what seemed strange at first by force of continued habit became a delight, and the sound of the voices cheered her loneliness and perplexity.

Meanwhile her parents grew old and feeble by reason of the tireless torment of their grief. The news of it was noised abroad and the elder sisters learned all that had befallen. Then grief and mourning straightway fell upon them, they left their homes and vied with one another in their haste to have sight and speech of their parents once again.

Now that very night Psyche's husband thus addressed her—for though she saw not her unknown spouse, her hands had felt him, and her ears could hear him:

"Sweet Psyche, my beloved wife, Fortune is turned cruel and threatens you with deadly peril. Watch, be most cautious and beware. Your sisters believe you dead and are distraught with grief. They will seek you and visit yonder crag. But if you should chance to hear their lamentations, answer them not, do not even look forth from the house, or you will drive me to bitter woe and yourself to utter destruction."

Psyche assented and promised she would do as her husband willed. But when he left her with the passing of night, the poor girl burst into weeping and consumed the whole day in tears and lamentation, crying that now in truth she was utterly undone; for she was kept a close captive within the walls of her luxurious prison and deprived of all human conversation. She might not even bring consolation to her sisters, who mourned her loss, nor even so much as set eyes on them. She would take no refreshment, she neither bathed nor ate but, weeping floods of tears, retired to sleep. After a little her husband came to her side somewhat earlier than his wont, caught her still weeping to his arms, and thus upbraided her:

"Was this your promise, my sweet Psyche? What can I, your husband, now hope or expect of you? Night and day you cease not from your anguish, not even when your husband clasps you to his heart. Come, now, be it as you will! Obey your heart, though its craving bring you nothing but harm. Only remember, when later you repent, that I warned you in good earnest."

But Psyche, when she heard these words, broke into entreaties, then threatened that she would slay herself, and at last prevailed upon her husband to grant her desire, that she might see her sisters, soothe their sorrows, and have speech with them. He yielded to the prayers of his new-wed bride, and further gave her leave to present her sisters with what she would of gold or jewels. But he warned her again and again, with words that struck terror to the soul, never to let her sisters persuade her by their ill counsels to inquire what her husband was like; if she yielded to the impious promptings of curiosity, she would exile herself forever from his embraces and from all the profusion of wealth that now was hers. She thanked her husband, and her soul was somewhat cheered. Then said she: "Sooner would I die a hundred deaths than be robbed of your sweet love. For whoever you are, I love you and adore you passionately. I love you as I love life itself. Compared with you Cupid's own self would be as nothing. But grant this boon also, I beseech you, and bid your servant, the wind of the West, to bring my sisters hither even as he bore me."

Then she rained on him beguiling kisses and endearing words and embraces that should constrain him to her will, and beside these allurements called him "husband sweet as honey, Psyche's life and love." Her husband yielded to the power and spell of her passionate murmurs, yielded against his will, and promised to do all; and then, as dawn drew near, he vanished from his wife's arms.

Meanwhile her sisters had made inquiry as to the situation of the crag where Psyche had been left, and they hastened to the spot. And when they were there, they began to beat their breasts and weep their eyes blind, until all the rocks and cliffs made answer, echoing to their ceaseless cries of grief. And now they began to call on their unhappy sister by name, till the piercing sound of their lamentable crying descended into the valley, and Psyche ran forth from the house in an ecstasy of trembling joy. "Why do you torment yourselves with these vain cries of woe?" she cried. "I whom you mourn am here. Cease your mournful cries and dry those cheeks that so long have streamed with tears, for even now you may embrace her whom you bewailed." Then, calling the West Wind, she told him of her husband's command, and he did at once as he was bidden and bore them down into the valley safe and sound on the wings of his soft breath. There the sisters embraced with eager kisses and took delight of one another, till the tears that they had dried welled forth again for very joy.

Then said Psyche: "Come now, enter with joy the

house that is my house and refresh your afflicted hearts with the presence of your own Psyche." So saying, she showed them all the riches of the golden house and made known to their ears the great household of voices that waited on her. Then she refreshed their weariness in the fairest of baths and with all the rich dainties of that celestial table till, their senses sated with the affluence of her heavenly wealth, they began to foster envy deep in their inmost hearts. At length one of them began to question her without ceasing, very closely and curiously, as to who was the lord of these celestial marvels, and who or of what sort was her husband. Nevertheless, Psyche would in no wise transgress her husband's ordinance or banish it from the secret places of her soul, but on the spur of the moment feigned that he was young and fair to view, his cheeks just shadowed with a beard of down, and that he was for the most part occupied with hunting among the mountains or along the countryside. Then, for fear that as their talk went on she might make some slip and betray her secret, she loaded them with gifts of wrought gold and jeweled necklaces and, calling the West Wind, committed them to his charge, to be carried back to the place from whence they came.

This done, those good sisters of hers returned home, and the gall of rising envy burned fierce within them, and they began to talk with one another often and loud and angrily. At last one of them spoke as follows: "Oh! cruel and unkind, unprofitable Fortune! Was this thy will that we, born of the same parents as Psyche, should endure so different a lot? Are we, the elder, who have been given to alien kings to be their handmaidens and banished from our home and country, to dwell like exiles far from our parents? And is she, the youngest, the last offspring of our mother's weary womb, to be the mistress of such treasure and have a god for husband? Why, she has not even the wit to know how to use such overflowing fortune rightly. Did you see, sister, how many and how rich are the jewels that lie in her house, what shining raiment and what glistening gems are there, and how wherever one goes one walks on gold, abundant gold? Why, if she has a husband as fair as she told us, there lives no happier woman in all the world. Woman, did I say? It may be that as his love increases, and his passion gathers its full force, the god whom she has wedded will make her also a goddess. In good truth she is a goddess already; such was her carriage, such her mien. The woman who has voices for handmaids, and can command even the winds, is aiming high and breathes a goddess's pride even now. Whereas I, poor wretch, have got a husband older than my father, balder than a pumpkin, and feebler than any child, and he keeps the whole house under lock and key."

The other took up the strain: "I am afflicted by a husband so doubled and bent with rheumatism that he never gives a thought to love. I have to rub his gnarled and stony fingers till my soft hands are blistered with his dirty bandages, and stinking lotion, and filthy plasters. I am more than an attentive wife, I am a hard-worked sick-nurse. You may bear your misfortunes with patience, or rather—for I will speak my mind plainly— with servility. As for me, I cannot any longer endure that such wealth and fortune should have fallen to one so unworthy. Remember with what pride and arrogance she dealt with us, with what boastful and extravagant ostentation she revealed her haughty temper! How scanty were the gifts she gave us from the vastness of her store, and how grudgingly she gave! And then, when she was tired of our presence, she had us bundled off and blown away upon a whistling breeze. If I am a woman and have a spark of life in me, I'll oust her from her fortune. And if, as I should suppose, our outrageous treatment rankles in your heart as it does in mine, let us both take resolute action. Let us not reveal our wrong to our parents or any other human being; let us not even seem to know anything of how she fares. It is enough that we have seen what we would gladly not have seen, without our declaring such glad news of her to our parents and all mankind. Those are not truly rich whose wealth is known to no man. She shall learn that we are her elder sisters and not her handmaids. But now let us go to our husbands and revisit our homes, which, even if they are poor, are at least respectable. Then, when we have taken earnest thought and formed our plans, let us return in our might to crush her pride."

This counsel of evil, where good should have been, pleased these wicked women. They hid all the precious gifts they had received and began with feigned grief to weep once more, rending their hair and tearing their faces, as indeed they deserved to be torn. Then, after hastily deterring their parents from further search by rekindling the burning anguish of their grief, they went swollen with mad rage to their own homes, there to contrive their wicked schemes against their innocent sister, yes, even to devise her death.

Meanwhile Psyche's unknown husband once more admonished her as he talked with her in the darkness of night: "Do you see," he said, "what great peril you are in? Fortune as yet but skirmishes at the outposts. Unless you are firm and cautious while she is yet far off, she will close hand to hand. Those false she-wolves are weaving some deep plot of sin against you, whose purpose is this: to persuade you to seek to know my face, which, as I have told you, if once you see, you will see no more. And so if hereafter those wicked ghouls come hither armed with their dark designs—and they will come, that I know—speak not at all with them, or if your simple, unsuspecting soul is too tender to endure that, at least neither give ear nor utterance to anything concerning your husband. For soon we shall have issue, and even now your womb, a child's as yet, bears a child like to you. If you keep my secret in silence, he shall be a god; if you divulge it, a mortal."

This news made Psyche glad; she lifted her head and rejoiced that she should be blest with a divine child. She exulted in the glory of the babe that should be, and was proud that she should be called a mother. Anxiously she counted the days as they increased and the months that passed by, and marveled as the promise grew. But now those two curses, those foul furies breathing adder's poison, hastened toward their goal and came sailing on their course with impious speed. Then her husband, who came not save for the brief space of night, warned Psyche once again: "The last day, the final peril is upon you; those hateful women, your kin and yet your foes, have put their armor on, have struck their camp, set the battle in array, and blown the trumpet blast; your monstrous sisters have drawn the sword and seek your life. Alas! sweetest Psyche, what calamities are upon us! Pity yourself and me, keep holy silence and save your house, your husband, yourself, and our young babe from the doom of ruin that lowers over them. Neither see nor hear those wicked women—sisters I may not call them—for they have conceived unnatural hate for you and have trodden underfoot the bonds of blood. Oh! take no heed when, like the Sirens, they stand forth upon the crag and make the cliffs echo with their fatal voices."

Psyche replied, her voice broken with tearful sobs: "Long since, I think, you have had proof of my fidelity and discretion. Not less, even now, will I show how steadfast is my soul. Only once more bid our servant the West Wind to perform his office. You have denied me sight of your holy form, grant me at least that I may see my sisters. By your locks that hang all round your brow, sweet as scent of cinnamon, by the soft delicate cheeks so like mine, by your bosom that burns with strange heat, I implore you, by my hopes that at least I may behold your face in the face of our babe, I beseech you, grant the pious prayer of my anguished entreaty, suffer me to enjoy the embraces of my sisters, and make the soul of Psyche, your votary, take new life for joy. I seek no more to see your face; not even the dark of night can be a hindrance to my joy, for I hold you in my arms, light of my life." With these words and soft embraces she charmed her husband to her will. Wiping away her tears with his own locks, he promised he would do as she desired and straightway departed before the light of dawning day.

The leagued conspirators, the two sisters, did not so much as set eyes on their parents but hastened with headlong speed to the crag. They tarried not for the coming of the wind that should bear them, but with presumptuous daring leapt forth into the abyss. But the West Wind forgot not the bidding of his king, though he had gladly done so, and caught them to the bosom of his breathing air and set them down upon the ground. They made no delay, but entered the house side by side; and there they that were Psyche's sisters only in name embraced their prey and, hiding beneath a cheerful mien the guile that was stored within their hearts as if it had been a treasure, spoke to her with these fawning words: "Psyche, you are no longer a child, no, you are even now a mother. Think what a joy to us you bear in your womb, with what delight you will make glad all our home. Ah! blessed are we who shall rejoice to nurse your golden babe, who if he match, as match he should, his parents' beauty, will be born a very Cupid."

Thus step by step with feigned love they wormed their way into their sister's heart. And straightway, when she had bidden them sit down, and had refreshed them from the weariness of their journey, and cheered them with steaming water at the bath, she feasted them royally in her banqueting hall on all those wondrous dainties and savory stews. She bade the harp sound, and its chords made melody; she bade the flute play, and its voice was heard; she bade the choir sing, and their chant pealed forth. The hearts of those who heard were made glad by all this ravishing music, although they saw no one. But yet not even the honeyed sweetness of those strains could allay the wicked purpose of those accursed women. They turned their speech to frame the snare that their guile had made ready, and with false words began to ask her what her husband was like, what was his family, what his rank. Then Psyche, in the utter simplicity of her heart, forgot her former tale and devised a new falsehood, and said that her husband came from the next province, had vast sums invested in business, and was middle-aged, his hair just grizzled with a few gray hairs. She spoke only for a moment on this matter and then, loading her sisters once more with costly gifts, sent them away in the chariot of the wind.

But, when the soft breath of the West had lifted them on high, and they were returning homeward, they began to speak thus one to the other: "What are we to say, sister, of so monstrous a falsehood as that which the poor fool told us? The first time her husband was a youth with manhood's first down upon his chin; now he is middle-aged in all the glory of white hairs. Who can he be whom so short a space of time has thus transformed into an old man? My sister, there are but two alternatives. Either the wretch lies, or else she does not know what her husband is like. Whichever of these explanations is true, it is our duty to cast her forth from that wealth of hers as soon as we may. But if she has never seen her husband's face, clearly she has married a god, and it is a god that she bears in her womb. Now, if she come to be called the mother of a baby god—which heaven forbid!

—I will get a noose and hang myself. Meanwhile, let us return home to our parents and devise some cunning deceit such as may suit our present discourse."

So hot with anger were they that they had scarcely a word of greeting for their parents and passed a sleepless and disturbed night. On the morrow these abandoned women hastened to the crag and swooped swiftly down as before under the protection of the wind. Then forcing a few tears from their eyes by rubbing their lids, they addressed their young sister with these crafty words: "Ah! you are happy, for you live in blessed ignorance of your evil plight and have no suspicion of your peril. But we cannot sleep for the care with which we watch over your happiness and are torn with anguish for your misfortunes. For we have learned the truth, and, since we are partners of your grief and hapless plight, we may not hide it from you. He that lies secretly by your side at night is a huge serpent with a thousand tangled coils; blood and deadly poison drip from his throat and from the cavernous horror of his gaping maw. Remember Apollo's oracle, how it proclaimed that you should be the bride of some fierce beast. Moreover, many a farmer, many a hunter of this neighborhood, and many of those who dwell round about have seen him as he returns from devouring his prey or swims in the shallows of the river. And all affirm that you will not much longer feast on such dainties or receive such loving service, but so soon as your time has come, he will devour you with the ripe fruit of your womb. The hour has now come when you must choose whether to believe your sisters, whose sole care is for your dear safety, to flee from death and live with us, free from all thought of peril, or find a grave in the entrails of a cruel monster. If the musical solitude of this fair landscape, if the joys of your secret love still delight you, and you are content to lie in the embraces of a foul and venomous snake, at least we, your loving sisters, have done our duty."

Poor Psyche, for she was a simple and gentle soul, was seized with terror at this melancholy news; she was swept beyond the bounds of reason, forgot all her husband's warnings and all her own promises. Headlong she fell into the deeps of woe, her limbs trembled, her face turned pale and bloodless, and in stumbling accents she stammered forth these scarcely articulate words: "Dearest sisters," she said, "you are true to your love for me, as is fitting. And I think that those who told you these things are not lying. For never have I seen my husband's face nor known at all whence he comes. Only at night I hear soft murmured words and endure the embraces of a husband who shuns the light and whose shape I know not. You say well that he is some strange beast, and I accept your words. For ever with stern speech he terrifies me from seeking to have sight of him, and threatens great woe to me should I strive curiously to look upon his face. Now, therefore, help me, if there be any succor you may bring to your sister in her hour of peril. For you will undo all your former good deeds, if you allow indifference to usurp the place of love."

Then since they had reached their sister's inmost heart and laid it bare to view, and its portals stood open wide, those evil women abandoned the secret stealth of their dark scheming, unsheathed the swords of guile, and invaded the timorous thoughts of the simple-hearted girl. Then said one of them: "Since the ties of birth bid us disregard all peril, if only we may save you, we will make known to you the course that long thought has revealed to us, the sole path that leads to safety. Take the sharpest of razors and whet it yet sharper by rubbing it softly against the palm of your hand, then hide it on the side of your couch where you are accustomed to lie. Take too some handy lantern, filled with oil and burning with a clear light, and place it beneath the cover of some vessel. Conceal all these preparations most carefully, and then, when he enters, trailing his moving coils, and climbs to his couch as is his custom, wait till he is stretched at full length and caught in the stupor of his first sleep, and his breathing tells you that his slumber is deep; then glide from the bed and barefoot, on tiptoe, moving soft with tiny steps, free the lantern from its prison in the blind dark. Let the light teach you how best to perform your glorious deed, then raise your right hand, put forth all your strength, and with the two-edged blade hew through the joint that knits the head and neck of the deadly serpent. Our aid shall not fail you. As soon as you have won safety by his death, we will hasten eagerly to your side, join hands with yours to bear away all your treasure, find you a wedlock worthy of your prayers, and unite you to a husband as human as yourself."

With these words they enflamed their sister's burning heart—for in truth her heart was all afire—and then left her, for they feared exceedingly to remain on the spot where so great a crime was to be done. As before, they were borne to the crag's top by the blast of the winged breeze, sped away in hasty flight, entered their ships, and departed.

✧

Psyche was left alone—and yet she was not at all alone, for the fierce furies that vexed her soul were ever with her. She tossed to and fro upon a tide of troubles vast as the sea. Her resolve was made and her heart fixed, yet as she strove to nerve her hands for the deed, her purpose failed her and was shaken, and she was distraught by the host of passions that were born of her anguish. Impatience, indecision, daring and terror, diffidence and anger, all strove within her, and, worst of all, in the same body she hated the beast and loved the husband. Yet as evening began to draw on to night, with precipitate haste she made all ready for her hideous crime. Now night was come and with it her husband; he caught her in his arms, kissed her, and sank into a deep sleep.

Then Psyche—for though flesh and spirit were weak and trembled, yet the fierce will of destiny gave her force—summoned all her strength, drew forth the lantern, and seized the razor; a sudden courage displaced the weakness of her sex. But as soon as the lamplight revealed the secrets of the couch, she saw the kindest and sweetest of all wild beasts, Amor himself, fairest of gods and fair even in sleep, so that even the flame of the lamp, when it beheld him, burned brighter for joy, and lightnings flashed from the razor's sacrilegious blade. But Psyche at the marvel of that sight was all dismayed, her soul was distraught, a sickly pallor came over her, fainting and trembling she sank to her knees and sought to hide the blade in her own heart. And this she would assuredly have done, had not the steel slipped from her rash hands for terror of so ill a deed. Weary and desperate, fallen from her health of mind and body, she gazed again and again upon the beauty of that divine face and her soul drew joy and strength. She beheld the glorious hair of his golden head streaming with ambrosia, the curling locks that strayed over his snow-white neck and crimson cheeks, some caught in a comely tangle, some hanging down in front, others behind; and before the lightnings of their exceeding splendor even the light of the lamp grew weak and faint. From the shoulders of the winged god sprang dewy pinions, shining like white flowers, and the topmost feathers, so soft and delicate were they, quivered tremulously in a restless dance, though all the rest were still. His body was smooth and very lovely and such as Venus might be proud to have borne. Before the feet of the god lay bow, quiver, and arrows, the kindly weapons of the great god. Psyche gazed on them with insatiate heart and burning curiosity, took them in her hands, and marveled at her husband's armory. Then, taking an arrow from the quiver, she tried its point against her thumb. But her hand trembled and pressed too hard upon it, till the point pricked too deep and tiny blood-drops bedewed the surface of her skin. So all unwitting, yet of her own doing, Psyche fell in love with Love. Then, as her passion for passion's lord burned her ever more and more, she cast herself upon him in an ecstasy of love, heaped wanton kiss on kiss with thirsty hastening lips, till she feared he might awake.

But even as her swooning spirit wavered in the ecstasy of such bliss, the lamp, whether foul falseness or guilty envy moved it, or whether it longed itself to touch and kiss so fair a body, sputtered forth from the top of its flame a drop of burning oil, which fell upon the god's right shoulder. Ah! rash, overbold lamp! Love's unworthy servant, thou burnest the very lord of fire, although surely thou dost owe thy being to some lover who devised thee that even by night he might have all his desire. For the god, when he felt the burning smart, leapt from the couch and, seeing his secret thus foully betrayed, tore himself from the kisses and embraces of his unhappy bride and flew away with never a word. But poor Psyche, even as he rose, caught hold of his right leg with both her hands, clung to him as he soared on high, and would not leave him, but followed him for the last time as he swept through the clouds of air, till at last overwearied she fell to earth.

But the god her lover left her not lying thus on earth, but flew to a cypress hard by, and from its lofty top spoke to her thus in accents of woe: "Ah! Psyche, simplehearted, I forgot the commands of my mother Venus, who bade me fire you with passion for some miserable abject man and yoke you in wedlock to him, and myself flew to your side that I might be your lover in his place. But this I did thoughtlessly, as now I know. For I, the far-famed archer, wounded myself with my own shafts, and made you my bride to win this reward—that you should think me a wild beast, and plot to hew off my head with blade of steel, that head where dwell these eyes that love you so dearly. Again and again I bade you beware of all that you have done, and in my love forewarned you. But those admirable women, your counselors, shall forthwith pay the penalty for their disastrous admonitions; you I will only punish thus—by flying from you." And with these words he spread his pinions and soared into the sky.

But Psyche, though she lay bowed to the earth, followed her husband's flight as far as sight could reach and tormented her soul with lamentation. When the beat of his wings had borne him far, and the depth of air had snatched him from her sight, she flung herself headlong from the brink of a river that flowed hard by. But the kindly stream feared for himself, and, to do honor to the god who kindles even waters with his fire, straightway caught her in his current and laid her unhurt upon a bank deep in flowering herbage. It chanced that at that moment Pan, the god of the countryside, sat on the river's brow with Echo, the mountain goddess, in his arms, teaching her to make melodious answer to sounds of every kind. Close by along the bank, goats wandered as they browsed and played wantonly as they plucked the river's leafage. The goat-footed god called Psyche to him gently, for she was bruised and swooning, and he knew moreover what had befallen her; and he assuaged her pain with these gentle words:

"Fair maiden, I am but a rude rustic shepherd, but long old age and ripe experience have taught me much. If I guess rightly (though men that are wise call it no guess, but rather divination), your weak and tottering steps, your body's exceeding pallor, your unceasing sighs, and still more your mournful eyes, tell me that you are faint from excess of love. Wherefore give ear to me and seek no more to slay yourself by casting yourself head-long down, nor by any manner of self-slaughter. Cease from your grief and lay aside your sorrow, and rather address Amor, the mightiest of gods, with fervent prayer and win him by tender submission, for he is an amorous and soft-hearted youth."

So spoke the shepherd god. Psyche made no answer, but worshiped the deity that had showed her the path of safety and went upon her way. When she had wandered no small way with weary feet, about close of day she came by a path she knew not to a certain town, where the husband of one of her sisters held sway. When she learned this, Psyche begged that her presence might be announced to her sister. She was led into the palace and there, when they had made an end of greeting and em-bracing one another, her sister asked her the reason of her coming. Psyche made answer thus: "You remember the counsel you gave me, when you urged me to take a two-edged razor and slay the wild beast that lay with me under the false name of husband, before my wretched body fell a victim to his voracious maw. But as soon as I took the lamp for my witness—for such, alas! was your counsel—and looked upon his face, I saw a won-drous, a celestial sight, the son of Venus, Amor himself, lying hushed in gentle slumber. Transported by the sight of so much joy, and distraught by my great gladness, my ecstasy was almost more than I could endure. But at that moment, by a cruel stroke of chance, the lamp spurted forth a drop of burning oil, which fell upon his shoulder. The pain wakened him from sleep, he saw me armed with fire and blade of steel and cried, 'In atonement for the foul crime you have purposed, begone from my couch and take with you what is yours. I will marry your sister'—and he mentioned your name—'with all due ritual.' So saying, he bade the West Wind blow me beyond the confines of the house."

Psyche had scarcely finished when her sister, goaded by the stings of mad lust and guilty envy, tricked her husband with a cunningly contrived lie, pretending that she had just received the news of her parents' death, and without more ado took ship and went to that same crag. And there, though it was no wind of the West that blew, yet, aflame with all the greed of blind hope, she cried: "Take me, Amor, a wife that is worthy of thee, and thou, wind of the West, bear up thy mistress." So saying, she hurled herself headlong in one mighty leap. But not even in death might she reach that happy place. For her limbs were tossed from rock to rock among the crags and torn asunder, and afterwards, as she deserved, she provided food for the birds and beasts who devoured her entrails. Such was the manner of her end.

Nor was the doom of Amor's second vengeance long delayed. For Psyche once more was led by her wandering feet to another city, where the other sister dwelt, as had dwelt the first. And like the first, she too was ensnared by Psyche's guile and, seeking in wicked rivalry to supplant her sister as the bride of Love, hastened to the crag, and perished by the same death.

Meanwhile, as Psyche wandered in search of Amor from people to people, he lay in his mother's chamber groaning for the pain of the wound that the lamp had dealt him. Then that white bird, the sea mew that swims over the surface of the waves oared by its wings, hastily plunged into the deep bosom of Ocean. There he found Venus, as she was bathing and swimming, and taking his stand by her told her that her son had been burned, that he was full of anguish at the wound's great pain and lay in peril of his life. Further he told her that the whole household of Venus had been brought into evil repute, and suffered all manner of railing, "because," said the bird, "both thou and he have retired from the world, he to revel with a harlot in the mountains, and thou, goddess, to swim the sea. And so there has been no pleasure, no joy, no merriment anywhere, but all things lie in rude unkempt neglect; wedlock and true friendship and parents' love for their children have vanished from the earth; there is one vast disorder, one hateful loathing and foul disregard of all bonds of love." Such were the words with which that garrulous and most inquisitive bird, as he chattered into Venus' ear, lacerated the reputation of her son. Venus was filled with anger and cried with a sudden cry: "And so that good son of mine has got a mistress! Come tell me, bird, my only faithful servant, what is the name of this woman who has thus distracted my son, a simple boy not yet promoted to the garb of manhood? Tell me, is it one of the Nymphs or Hours? Or is it one of the Muses' choir, or one of my own attendant Graces?"

The loquacious bird had no thought of silence. "Mistress," he replied, "I know not who she is. I think, however, if my remembrance does not play me false, that he

was head over ears in love with a girl called Psyche."
Then Venus in her indignation cried yet louder still:
"What! he loves Psyche, the supplanter of my beauty
and the rival of my fame! Why, the young scamp must
think me his procuress, for it was I who showed him the
girl, and it was through me that he came to know her!"

Shrieking such words as these, she emerged from the
sea and straightway sought her golden chamber. And
finding the boy lying sick even as she had heard, she
railed loudly at him as soon as she reached the door of
the room: "Truly your behavior is most honorable and
worthy of your birth and your own good name, first to
trample your mother's, or rather your queen's, bidding
underfoot, to refuse to torment my enemy with base desires, and then actually to take her to your own wanton
embraces, mere boy as you are, so that I must endure my
enemy as my daughter-in-law! Oh! you seducer, you
worthless boy, you matricidal wretch! You think, no
doubt, that you alone can have offspring and that I am
too old to bear a child. I would have you know that I
will bear a far better son than you have been. No, to
give the insult a sharper sting, I will adopt one of my
own young slaves, give him your feathers and your
flames, your bow and arrows and all the trappings I
gave you for use far other than that which you have
made of them. For nothing of all that went to make up
your accouterments came from your father's estate! You
have been badly trained from your babyhood till now;
you have sharp talons and have often beaten your elders
in the most irreverent manner, why, you have robbed
your own mother, yes, you rob me daily, you unnatural

son! You have often stricken me, you treat me with scorn as being a widow, and show not the least reverence for your stepfather, the greatest and bravest of all warriors. Why, you have even provided him with paramours, because you are angry with my love for him! But I will make you rue those tricks and your marriage shall be as bitter gall in your mouth. But what shall I do now to avenge my mockery? Where shall I turn? How shall I restrain this foul little eft? Shall I seek aid from my foe Sobriety, whom I have so often offended to satisfy his whims? No, I cannot endure the thought of speaking to a creature so rude and unkempt. On the other hand, my vengeance is not to be despised, from whatever source it may come. I will seek her aid and hers alone. She shall punish that young ne'er-do-well right soundly, empty his quiver and blunt his arrows, unstring his bow and extinguish the flames of his torch, yes, and apply even sharper remedies to his body itself. Only then shall I feel wrong appeased, when she has clipped his hair close, that hair to which I with my own hands gave its sheen of gold, and when she has shorn away those wings which I steeped in nectar as he lay in my bosom."

So speaking, she flung out of doors in bitter anger, and ah! how bitter the wrath of Venus can be! But Ceres and Juno straightway met her and, seeing her face thus distorted with passion, asked why she had imprisoned all the charm of her flashing eyes with so fierce a frown. She answered: "It is well you have met me! For my heart is all on fire, and I should have done some violence. But go, I pray you, with all your might seek out that wretch, Psyche, who has made off as if on wings.

For you cannot be ignorant of the shame that has befallen my house, nor of the deeds of my unspeakable son."

Then, although they knew well what had come to pass, they strove to soothe the wrath of Venus. "What great crime," they asked, "has your son committed that you should denounce his pleasures so fiercely and seek to kill her whom he loves? Even if he has smiled not unwillingly on a charming girl, is that a crime? Don't you know that he is a man and young? Or have you forgotten the number of his years? Or do you think he must always be a boy merely because he carries his years so fairly? And must you, his mother, a sensible woman too, always be prying curiously into your son's amusements, blaming him for a wanton, taunting him with his loves, and denouncing your own arts and your own charms that live again in your fair son? Who among gods and men will permit you to sow passions broadcast among the peoples of the earth, while you forbid your own household the charms of love, and debar them from all enjoyment of woman's foibles, an enjoyment that is open to all the world?"

Thus the goddesses, in fear of Amor's arrow, gladly took up his defense and flattered him even in his absence. But Venus, indignant that her wrongs should be treated with such ridicule, passed them by and departed in the opposite direction, seeking the sea with hasty steps.

Meanwhile Psyche wandered hither and thither in restless agitation. Night and day she sought her husband and her heart could not find rest. And more and more she yearned, if the tender blandishments of a wife might not allay his anger, at least to appease him with the prayers of a slave. At last she saw a temple on the crest of a high mountain. "How do I know," she said, "that my lord may not dwell yonder?" And there she hastened, for hope and desire lent wings to her feet, though they were fainting beneath her for very weariness of her unending toil. And now she had nimbly surmounted the high ridge and entered and approached the sacred couch. There she saw sheaves of wheat piled in a heap or twined into garlands; sheaves too of barley were there, and sickles and all the implements of the reaper's calling. But all lay at random, confused and uncared for, as though they had been cast idly down by the reapers' hands in the heat of noon. Psyche separated them all with care and arranged them in due order, each in its separate place; for she thought that she ought not to neglect the shrines or ceremonies of any god, but rather appeal to the kindness and pity of all. While she was thus engaged with anxious industry, kindly Ceres came upon her and straightway cried aloud, "Is it you, poor Psyche? Venus in the madness of her heart tracks your steps anxiously through all the world, seeking that she may mete out to you the most cruel of punishments, and eager to avenge her wrong with all the might of her godhead. And yet do you now watch thus over my offerings, and have you thought for your own safety?"

Then Psyche cast herself down on the ground before her, bedewing the goddess's feet with floods of tears and sweeping the ground with her hair. And with manifold entreaties she besought that she might win pardon. "By thy right hand that bringeth fruit to the earth, by the glad rites of harvest, by the silent mysteries of thy sacred arks, by the winged chariots drawn by the dragons that serve thee, by the furrows of Sicilian fields, by the rav- isher's chariot and the imprisoning earth, by the deep abyss where the lightless wedlock of Proserpine was cele- brated, by the joyous return to the light when thou hadst found thy daughter, and by all else that the shrine of Attic Eleusis shrouds in silence, I beseech thee, succor the soul of helpless Psyche, thy suppliant. Suffer me to lie hid, if only for a few short days, amid yonder heap of sheaves, that the wild anger of that mighty goddess may be assuaged by lapse of time, or at least that I may find a brief space of rest and refreshment for my strength that my long toil hath broken."

Ceres answered: "Your tearful prayers awaken my pity and I long to aid you, but I may not quarrel with one who is my kinswoman. Moreover, I am bound to her also by old ties of friendship, and she has a good heart after all. And so you must leave my temple without more ado, and count it for the best that I have not kept you here, nor given you my protection."

This unlooked-for repulse doubled Psyche's affliction, and she turned back from the temple. As she went she saw in a twilight grove within a deep valley a temple built of cunning workmanship, and since she wished to leave no path to fairer hope untried, however doubtful it might be, but rather to implore the aid of every god, she approached the sacred portals. She saw there precious gifts and cloths embroidered with letters of gold hang- ing from the boughs of trees or fastened to the door- posts. And all these bore witness to the name of the goddess to whom they had been dedicated in gratitude for boons received at her hand. Then Psyche sank to her knee and, casting her hands about the altar, still warm with sacrifice, wiped away her tears and made her prayer:

"Sister and bride of mighty Jove, whether thou holdest thine ancient home at Samos, which alone hath glory from thy birth, thine infant wailing, and thy nurture; or whether thou hauntest thy rich home in lofty Carthage, that honors thee as the maid that came down from heaven borne on the lion's back; or rulest thou over the glorious walls of Argos by the banks of Inachus, who proclaims thee bride of the Thunderer and queen of goddesses, thou whom all the East worships as Zygia and all the West hails as Lucina, be thou to me in my great need Juno the Savior, and free me from the fear of imminent peril; for the toils I have endured are great and I am very weary. Aye, and I know that, even uncalled, thou aidest mothers in peril when their time is near."

So prayed she, and forthwith Juno revealed herself to her in all the august majesty of her godhead, and straightway said: "Right gladly, by my honor, I swear it, right gladly would I grant your prayers. But for very shame I may not aid you against the will of Venus, my son's wife, whom I have ever loved as a daughter. Moreover, I am prevented by the laws forbidding harborage to others' runaway slaves, save only with their master's consent."

This second shipwreck of her fortunes filled Psyche with terror. She had sought her winged husband all in vain and, despairing utterly of safety, thus brooded within herself: "What help now may I seek for the healing of my woes, since even these goddesses, for all their good will, may not lift their voice in my defense? Whither now may I turn, that am caught in so vast a snare? What house, what darkness may hide me safe from great Venus' inevitable eyes! Come then, take heart of grace! Your poor hopes are shattered. Renounce them boldly and yield of your own free will to your mistress, and assuage the fierce onset of her wrath by submission, late though it be. Who knows but you may even find the husband you have sought so long, there in his mother's house!" And so she made ready for the uncertain issue of her submission, or rather for certain death, and meditated how she should begin her entreaties.

Venus, meanwhile, had abandoned all attempts to search her out on earth and sought the skies. She bade her chariot be prepared, the chariot that Vulcan had wrought for her of gold, and finished carefully with subtle art, and given her as a marriage gift, before they passed the threshold of the bridal chamber. It shone where the artist's file had thinned the metal away, and the very loss of the gold had made it more precious. Four white doves, out of all the many that nested round their mistress's bedchamber, appeared and, hopping gaily forth and writhing their painted necks, entered the jeweled yoke; their mistress mounted the car, and they flew forth bearing her on their way with joy. Sparrows wantoned in the air with twittering harmony, as they attended the chariot of the goddess, and every manner of sweet songbird proclaimed her coming with the melodious music of their honeyed strains. The clouds yielded before her path, heaven opened to his daughter, and the heights of air welcomed her with joy; nor had the musical servants of mighty Venus any fear of pouncing eagle or greedy hawk.

Then she turned her course to Jove's royal castle and, superb even in her supplications, demanded that Mercury, god of the ringing voice, should be placed at her disposal to lend her his aid. Jove's dark brow nodded assent, and straightway Venus descended from heaven in an ecstasy of joy and addressed Mercury, who went with her, in these earnest words: "Arcadian brother, you know that your sister Venus has never done anything without the aid of Mercury, and you cannot but be aware how long I have searched in vain for that handmaiden of mine who hides from me. There is nothing left for me but to employ you as my herald and publish a reward for her discovery. See then that you perform my behest with speed and set forth clearly the marks by which she may be known, that no one who has wickedly and unlawfully taken upon him to conceal her may plead ignorance as an excuse." So saying, she gave him a handbill containing Psyche's name and all else that was necessary. This done, she went home.

Mercury did not neglect to do as he was bidden. For he sped far and wide, visiting all the peoples of the earth, and thus performed the task of proclamation with which he had been entrusted: "If any man can stay the flight or point out the hiding place of a runaway princess, handmaid of Venus, answering to the name of Psyche, let him meet Mercury, who makes this proclamation, behind the Murcian Pyramids, and he shall receive as the reward of his information seven sweet kisses from Venus' own lips and one yet more honeyed than the rest from the tip of her sweet tongue."

When Mercury delivered his proclamation in this wise, a wild desire seized all mankind, and they vied with one another in the hope of winning so marvelous a reward. This circumstance more than all else finally banished every thought of further delay from Psyche's soul. And as she was already approaching the doors of her mistress, one of Venus' servants, Habit by name, met her and at once cried with all the strength of her voice: "So at last you have come to understand who is your mistress, you worthless slut! Or do you still pretend not to know what trouble we have had in looking for you? It would be in keeping with the rest of your effrontery if you did. But it is lucky you have fallen into my hands. Hell has you in its claws now, and you shall pay bitterly for your disobedience, now without more ado." Then without a moment's hesitation she thrust her hand into Psyche's hair and dragged her after her.

Psyche made no resistance, but was led into the house and brought into the presence of Venus. The goddess no sooner beheld her than she burst into a wild laugh, such as men will utter when mad with wrath; then shaking her head and scratching her right ear, she cried: "So, at length you have thought fit to come and greet your mother-in-law? Or have you come to visit your husband, who is in danger of his life, thanks to the wound you gave him? But you need not be frightened!

I will give you such a welcome as a good daughter-in-law deserves." Then "Where," she cried, "are my hand-maidens Trouble and Sorrow?" They were summoned, and Venus handed over Psyche to their charge, so that they might torture her. In obedience to their mistress's command, they scourged poor Psyche with whips and racked her with other torments, and then once more brought her into the presence of their mistress.

Then Venus laughed loud once again and said: "Behold, she thinks to move me with pity because she is big with child and the time is near when the fair fruit of her womb shall make me a happy grandmother. Truly, I am highly blessed that I should be called a grand-mother, though yet in the flower of my age, and that the son of a vile serving-wench should be known as Venus' grandchild! But I am a fool to call him her son. He is no true son, for the parties to the marriage were not of equal birth, while the wedding took place in a country house unwitnessed and without his father's con-sent. It cannot therefore be regarded as legitimate, and the child will be born a bastard, at least if we allow you to become a mother at all."

So saying, she flew upon her, tore her clothes in many places, dishevelled her hair, buffeted her about the head, and beat her cruelly. Then, taking corn and barley and millet and poppy seed and chick peas and lentils and beans, all jumbled and confused in one heap, she said to her: "I cannot conceive that any serving-wench as hideous as yourself could find any means to attract lovers save by making herself their drudge; wherefore now I my-self will make trial of your worth. Sort that disordered heap of seeds, place each kind of grain apart in its own place, and see that you show me the work completed before the evening."

Having thus assigned her this vast heap of seeds, the goddess departed to a marriage feast. But Psyche never put a hand to that disordered and inextricable mass, but sat in silent stupefaction, overwhelmed by the vastness of the task. Then the ant, the little ant, that dweller in the fields, understanding the difficulty of her huge task, pitied the sorrow of the great god's bride and, abhorring the cruelty of her mother-in-law, ran nimbly hither and thither and summoned and gathered all the host of ants that dwelt around. "Pity," it cried, "O ye nimble nurslings of earth, the mother of all; pity a lovely girl, the spouse even of Love himself. Be prompt and swift and aid her in her hour of need!" Thereupon, wave upon wave, the six-footed hosts rushed to the rescue, and one by one, with the utmost zeal, separated the whole heap, grain by grain. And after they had parted and distributed the several grains, each after their kind, they vanished swiftly from sight.

And now at nightfall Venus returned from the wedding feast, heavy with wine and sweet with balsam scents and all her body bound about with shining roses. And when she saw with what marvelous diligence the task had been performed, she cried: "This is not your doing, vile wretch, nor the work of your hands, but the work of him whose heart you won to your own hurt, yes, and to his hurt also." Then, flinging her a crust of common bread, she departed to her couch. Meanwhile Amor was kept under close ward in the inner part of the house within the four walls of his own chamber, partly that he might not inflame his wound by the perversity of his wanton passions, partly that he might not meet his beloved. And so those two lovers dragged out the night of woe beneath the same roof, but sundered and apart. But when Aurora had just begun to ride forth in the sky, Venus called Psyche to her and thus addressed her: "Do you see that grove that fringes the long banks of the gliding stream, whose deep eddies come rushing down from yonder mountain? There wander sheep whose fleeces shine with hue of gold, and no man guards them as they graze. I bid you take a wisp from the wool of their precious fleece as best you may and bring it to me with speed."

Psyche arose willingly, not indeed that she might perform her task, but that she might find rest from her woes by casting herself down a cliff that overhung the river. But from the river's bed a green reed, nurse of sweet music, breathed on by some breath divine, with gentle murmur whispered forth this melodious prophecy: "Psyche, racked though thou art by so many a woe, pollute not my sacred waters by slaying thyself thus miserably, nor at this hour approach those terrible sheep. For they borrow fierce heat from the blazing sun and wild frenzy maddens them, so that with sharp horns and foreheads hard as stone, and sometimes even with venomous bites, they vent their fury in the destruction of men. But till the heat of the noonday sun has assuaged its burning, and the beasts are lulled to sleep by the soft river breeze, thou canst hide thee beneath yonder lofty plane tree, which drinks of the river water even as I. And, when once the sheep have abated their madness and allayed their anger, go shake the leaves of yonder grove, and thou shalt find the golden wool clinging here and there to crooked twigs."

Thus did that kind and simple-hearted reed teach Psyche in her deep distress how she might win to safety. She listened with an attention which she had no cause to regret and thus instructed made no delay, but observed all the bidding of the reed, stole the soft yellow gold with easy theft, and returned to Venus with her bosom full of it. And yet she won no approval from her mistress for having overcome the peril of her second task. For Venus, with a frown upon her brow and a bitter smile upon her lips, said: "I am well aware who was the secret author of this deed no less than the last. But now I will put you to a shrewd trial that I may know whether you have a stout heart and prudence beyond the prudence of woman. Do you see the high mountain peak that crowns yonder lofty cliff, wherefrom the swarthy waves of a black stream flow down till, caught in the neighboring valley's walled abyss, they flood the Stygian swamps and feed the hoarse streams of Cocytus? Go, draw me icy water even from where on the high summit the fountain's farthest waves well forth, and bring it to me with all speed in this small urn." So saying, she gave her a small jar carved out of crystal, and threatened yet more cruel torments if she failed.

Then Psyche with swift steps sought the topmost height of the mountain, sure that there at least, if all else failed, she could put an end to her miserable existence. But as soon as she reached the slopes near the aforesaid peak she perceived how vast and difficult was her task, and how fraught with death. For it was a rock of measureless height, rough, slippery, and inaccessible, and from jaws that gaped in its midst it vomited forth a hideous stream that, from the very point where it burst from the hollows of a deep slanting cavern and fell over the rock's sloped face, had worn out a narrow channel for its path and, thus concealed, rushed secretly into the neighboring valley. To right and left from crannies in the crag there crept forth fierce dragons, with long craning necks and eyes sworn to unwinking wakefulness, whose pupils keep watch forever and shrink not from the light. And even the very waters had voices that forbade approach. For they cried "Hence!" and "What dost thou? Have a care!" and "What wouldst thou? Beware!" and "Fly!" and lastly "Thou art doomed to die!" Psyche felt herself turned to stone by the impossibility of her task. Though she was present in the body, her senses had flown far away from her and, quite overwhelmed by such vast inevitable peril, she lacked even the last solace of tears.

But the anguish of her innocent soul was not unmarked by the grave eyes of kindly Providence, for the royal bird of highest Jove suddenly spread both his pinions and came to her with timely aid, even the eagle, the ravisher, mindful of the ancient service rendered Jove when at Love's bidding he had swept from earth the Phrygian boy who is his cupbearer. He honored Love's godhead in the woes of his bride and, leaving the shining paths of the high vault of heaven, swooped past Psyche's face and thus began: "Dost thou, simple-hearted and all unversed in such labors, hope to have power to steal or even touch so much as one drop of that most holy and also most cruel fountain? Thou hast surely heard tell, even if thou hast never read, that even the gods and Jove himself dread yonder Stygian waters, and even as you mortals swear by the divinity of the gods, so the gods swear by the majesty of Styx. But come, give me that urn!" Straightway he seized it and caught it to his body; then poised on the vast expanse of his beating pinions, swiftly he oared his way among the fierce jaws of teeth and the forked tongues of dragons that flickered to left and right. The waters denied him access and bade him depart ere he took some hurt, but he feigned that he sought them at Venus' bidding and was her servant. Whereupon they suffered him to approach somewhat less grudgingly. So he took of the water and Psyche received the full urn with joy and bore it back with all speed to Venus.

Yet not even then could she appease the will of the frenzied goddess. For she threatened her with shameful torments yet worse and greater than before and thus addressed her with a baleful smile upon her lips: "In truth, I believe you are some great and potent sorceress, so nimbly have you obeyed my hard commands! But you must do me yet this one service, sweetheart. Take this casket"—and with the words she gave it—"and straightway descend to the world below and the ghastly halls of Orcus himself. There present the casket to Proserpine and say, 'Venus begs of thee to send her a small portion of thy beauty, such at least as may suffice for the space of one brief day. For all her beauty is worn and perished through watching over her sick son.' But see that you come back with all speed, for I must anoint myself with it before I go to heaven's theater."

Then Psyche felt more than ever that her fortune was come to its last ebb, and knew that all veil of pretense was laid aside, and that she was being driven to swift destruction. Well might she think so! For she was constrained with her own feet to tread the way to Tartarus and the spirits of the dead. She hesitated no longer, but went to a certain high tower that she might throw herself headlong from it. For thus she thought most swiftly and with greatest honor to descend to the world below.

But the tower suddenly broke forth into speech and cried: "Why, poor wretch, seekest thou to slay thyself by casting thyself headlong down? And why rashly dost thou faint before this task, the last of all thy perils? For if once the breath be severed from thy body, thou wilt assuredly go to the depths of Tartarus, but thou shalt in no wise have power to return thence. Give ear to me. Lacedaemon, a famous city of Achaea, is not far distant. Do thou seek Taenarus, that lies upon its borders hidden in a trackless wild. There is the vent of Dis, and through its gaping portals is shown a path where no man treads. Cross the threshold and launch thyself upon the path and forthwith thou shalt find a straight way to the very palace of Orcus. Yet thou must not go empty-handed through the gloom, but must bear in both thy hands cakes kneaded of pearl barley and mead, and in thy mouth itself thou must bear two coins. And when thou hast traversed a good part of thy deathly journey, thou shalt meet a lame ass bearing wood and with him a lame driver who will ask thee to hand him a few twigs that have fallen from the load. But do thou speak never a word, but pass on thy way in silence. And forthwith thou shalt come to the river of the dead, where Charon hath charge and asks the ferryman's toll before he conveys the traveler to the farther shore in his seamy bark. For avarice lives even among the dead, nor will Charon, or even the great god that is lord of hell, do anything unpaid; but the poor man when he dies must seek for journey money, and if there be no coin of bronze to hand, no one will ever suffer him to breathe his last. Thou must give this filthy graybeard by way of toll one of the coins which thou shalt take with thee. But remember, he must take it with his own hand from thy mouth. Likewise, as thou crossest the sluggish river, a dead man that is floating on the surface will pray thee, raising his rotting hands, to take him into thy boat. But be thou not moved with pity for him, for it is not lawful. And when thou hast crossed the river and gone a little way farther, old weaving women, as they weave their web, will beg thee lend them the aid of thy hands for a little. But thou must not touch the web; it is forbidden. For all these snares and many others spring from Venus' crafty designs against thee, that thou mayest let fall at least one of the cakes from thy hands. But think not the loss of that worthless piece of barley paste matters but little; for if thou lose but one, thou shalt lose with it the light of day. For there is a huge hound with three vast heads, wild and terrible, that bays with thunderous throat at the dead, though they are past all hurt that he might do them. Terrifying them with vain threats, he keeps sleepless watch before the very threshold of Prosperine's dark halls and guards the empty house of Dis. Bridle his rage by leaving him a cake to prey upon, and thou shalt pass him by with ease, and forthwith enter the very house of Proserpine. She shall welcome thee with kindly courtesy, bidding thee sit down and partake of a rich feast. But do thou sit upon the ground, and ask for coarse bread and eat it. Then tell wherefore thou hast come, take whatsoever shall be given thee and, returning back, buy off the hound's rage with the remaining cake. Then give the greedy mariner the coin thou hadst kept back and, when thou hast crossed the river, retrace thy former steps till thou behold once more yonder host of all the stars of heaven. But I bid thee, above all, beware that thou seek not to open or look within the casket which thou bearest, or turn at all with over-curious eyes to view the treasure of divine beauty that is concealed within."

Thus did that far-seeing tower perform its task of prophecy. And Psyche tarried not, but went to Taenarus and, duly taking the coins and the cakes, ran down the path to the underworld, passed by the decrepit donkey-driver in silence, paid the river's toll to the ferryman, disregarded the prayer of the floating dead, spurned the crafty entreaties of the weaving women and, after she had lulled the dread fury of the hound by giving him a cake to devour, entered the house of Proserpine. And though her hostess offered her a soft chair and dainty food she would have none of them, but sat lowly at her feet, content with common bread, and delivered the message with which Venus had entrusted her. Straightway the casket was filled and sealed in secret. Psyche took it in her hands, silenced the hound's barking maw with the second cake, paid the second coin to the ferryman, and, returning from the world below far more nimbly than she had descended, regained the shining daylight and worshiped it with adoration.

But then, although she was in haste to bring her task to its conclusion, her mind was overwhelmed with rash curiosity. "Oh! what a fool am I," she said, "for I carry the gift of divine beauty and yet sip not even the least drop therefrom, even though by so doing I should win the grace of my fair lover." With the words she unclasped the casket. But there was no beauty therein, nor anything at all save a hellish and truly Stygian sleep which, so soon as it was set free by the removal of the lid, rushed upon her and poured over all her limbs in a thick cloud of slumber. She fell in the very path where she stood, and the sleep possessed her where she fell. There she lay motionless, no better than a sleeping corpse.

❖

But the god Amor, who was recovering from his wound, which had now healed, unable to endure the long absence of his sweet Psyche, slipped through the lofty window of the bedchamber where he was confined and, since his wings had been refreshed by their long rest, flew forth swifter than ever and hastened to the side of his beloved Psyche. Carefully he wiped the sleep from off her and confined it in the casket, its former receptacle. Then waking Psyche with a harmless prick from one of his arrows, he said: "My poor child, your curiosity had almost brought you to destruction yet a second time. But meanwhile make haste to perform the task with which my mother charged you; I will see to the rest." So saying, her lover rose lightly upon his wings, and Psyche with all speed bore the gift of Proserpine to Venus.

Meanwhile Amor, pale-faced and devoured with very great love, and fearing the sudden earnestness that had possessed his mother, had recourse to his old tricks. Swift-winged he soared to heaven's farthest height, besought great Jove to aid him, and set forth his case. Thereupon Jove pinched Amor's cheek, raised his hand to his lips, kissed it, and thus made answer: "My son and master, you have never shown me the honor decreed me by the gods, but with continued blows have wounded this heart of mine whereby the laws of the elements and the motions of the stars are ordered, and have brought shame upon me by often causing me to fall into earthly lusts; you have hurt my good name and fame by tempting me to base adulteries in defiance of public law and order, why, you have even led me to transgress the Julian law itself; you have made me foully to disfigure my serene countenance by taking upon me the likeness of serpents, fire, wild beasts, birds, and cattle of the field. Yet, notwithstanding, mindful of my clemency and remembering that you have grown up in my arms, I will grant you all your suit on one condition. You shall be on your guard against your rivals and, if there be on earth a girl of surpassing beauty, shall repay my present bounty by making her mine."

Having thus spoken, he bade Mercury forthwith summon all the gods to an assembly and make proclamation that, if any one absented himself from the council of the heavenly ones, he should be fined ten thousand pieces. The fear of this caused heaven's theater promptly to be filled, and Jove, towering above the assembly on his high throne, thus gave utterance: "Gods whose names are written in the Muses' register, you all know right well, I think, that my own hands have reared the stripling whom you see before you. I have thought fit at last to set some curb upon the wild passions of his youthful prime. Long enough he has been the daily talk and scandal of all the world for his gallantries and his manifold vices. It is time that he should have no more occasion for his lusts; the wanton spirit of boyhood must be enchained in the fetters of wedlock. He has chosen a maiden, and robbed her of her honor. Let him keep her, let her be his forever, let him enjoy his love and hold Psyche in his arms to all eternity." Then, turning to Venus, he added: "And you, my daughter, be not downcast, and have no fear your son's marriage with a mortal will shame your lofty rank and lineage. For I will see to it that it shall be no unworthy wedlock, but lawful and in accordance with civil law." Then straightway he bade Mercury catch up Psyche and bring her to heaven. This done, he offered her a goblet of ambrosia and said: "Psyche, drink of this and be immortal. Then Amor shall never leave your arms, but your marriage shall endure forever."

Forthwith a rich nuptial banquet was set forth. The bridegroom reclined on the couch of honor holding

Psyche to his heart. So, too, Jove lay by the side of Juno his spouse, and all the gods took their places in order. Then the shepherd boy that is his cupbearer served Jove with a goblet of nectar, which is the wine of the gods, and Liber served the others, while Vulcan cooked the dinner. The Hours made all things glow red with roses and other flowers, the Graces sprinkled balsam, and the Muses made melody with tuneful voices. Apollo accompanied his lyre with song, fair Venus danced with steps that kept time to the sweet music played by the orchestra she had provided; for the Muses chanted in chorus or blew the flute, while Satyr and young Pan played upon the pipe of reed. Thus did Psyche with all solemnity become Amor's bride, and soon a daughter was born to them: in the language of mortals she is called Pleasure.

THE COMMENTARY

*The Psychic Development
of the Feminine*

FORENOTE

IN our interpretation we have not spoken of Cupid and Psyche as in Apuleius' text, which thus mixes Roman and Greek elements, but of Eros and Psyche, and we have uniformly translated the name back into its Greek form. It is not out of philological pedantry, which would be particularly unsuited to this text, that we have transposed the names of the gods into Greek. From a literary standpoint, there is no doubt that the frivolous late-Roman pantheon surrounding Psyche constitutes a part of the tale's charm. But in our interpretation, which stresses mythical motifs, it seems more fitting to speak of the Eleusinian mysteries of Demeter, rather than of Ceres, and to call the Argive goddess Hera rather than Juno. Still more important, it is Aphrodite and not Venus, who in our eyes is associated with the Great Goddess, and in the myth Psyche's lover and husband is the mighty, primordial god Eros, and not Amor or Cupid—the cunning little cherub known to us even from ancient works of art.

E.N.

The Psychic Development
of the Feminine

T HE tale of Eros and Psyche falls into five parts—
the introduction, the marriage of death, the act,
the four tasks, the happy end—and we shall follow this division in our interpretation. Psyche, the sub-
limely beautiful princess, is worshiped as a goddess.
Men neglect the cult of Aphrodite and undertake pil-
grimages to Psyche. This arouses the deadly jealousy of
Aphrodite, who bids her son Eros to avenge her and to
destroy Psyche by making her fall in love with the
"vilest of men."

With all her beauty, Psyche is unloved. In order to
obtain a husband for her, her father consults the oracle
and receives this terrible answer:

> On some high crag, O king, set forth the maid,
> In all the pomp of funeral robes arrayed.
> Hope for no bridegroom born of mortal seed,
> But fierce and wild and of the dragon breed.
> He swoops all-conquering, borne on airy wing,
> With fire and sword he makes his harvesting;
> Trembles before him Jove, whom gods do dread,
> And quakes the darksome river of the dead.

In obedience to the oracle's command, the unhappy
parents abandon Psyche to the marriage of death with
the monster. Surprisingly, Psyche is not slain; carried
off by Zephyr, she enters upon a paradisaical life with the
invisible husband, Eros, who has chosen her for his wife.

But her envious sisters break in upon this idyll of Psyche and Eros. Despite Eros' warnings, Psyche gives ear to her sisters and decides to surprise the monster (for her sisters have represented her husband as such) by night and to kill him. In the next part Psyche, disobeying Eros' command, looks upon him by the light of her lamp. She recognizes Eros as a god, but a scalding drop of oil awakens him, so that, just as he had warned her, she loses him at the same time. There follow Psyche's search for her lost lover, her struggle with Aphrodite's wrath, her performance of the labors imposed on her by the goddess. The contest ends with the defeat of Psyche, who opens Persephone's box and falls into a deathlike sleep. In the final chapter Psyche is redeemed by Eros and received on Olympus as his immortal wife.

The tale begins with the conflict between Psyche and Aphrodite. Psyche's beauty is so great that she is worshiped as a goddess. It is said among mortals that the goddess, "who sprang from the blue deep of the sea and was born from the spray of the foaming waves, had deigned to manifest her godhead to all the world and was dwelling among earthly folk." But still more offensive to Aphrodite is the profoundly symbolic belief "that heaven had rained fresh procreative dew, and earth, not sea, had brought forth as a flower a second Venus in all the glory of her maidenhood." According to this strange belief, Psyche was no longer an incarnation of Aphrodite, a notion that the goddess might conceivably have tolerated; instead she was "a second Aphrodite," newly begotten and newly born. Unquestionably this "new belief" contains an allusion to the birth of

Aphrodite, who, according to the myth, was created from the severed phallus of Uranus, which had fallen into the sea. Psyche, by contrast, the "new Aphrodite," is held to have been born of the earth impregnated by a drop of heaven's procreative dew.

It will become evident in the course of our discussion that this "new belief" is not the product of any arbitrary interpretation on our part but touches the very core of the myth. The conflict between Aphrodite and Psyche at the very beginning of the tale shows this to be the central motif.

The birth of Psyche is a critical event in human history, as is shown by the radical transformation of man's relation to Aphrodite. It corresponds exactly to the cry "Great Pan is dead!" that rang out at the end of antiquity. "And now many a mortal journeyed from far and sailed over the great deeps of ocean, flocking to see the wonder and glory of the age. Now no man sailed to Paphos or Cnidos, or even to Cythera, that they might behold the goddess Venus; her rites were put aside, her temples fell to ruin, her sacred couches were disregarded, her ceremonies neglected, her images uncrowned, her altars desolate and foul with fireless ashes. It was to a girl men prayed. . . ."

In reaction to all this, Aphrodite, as a "class-conscious" goddess, works herself up into a great rage. She, the "first parent of created things, the primal source of all the elements," to be treated thus! Her name "that dwells in the heavens" has been "dragged through the earthly muck." Her vanity is wounded, she is a jealous woman, thirsting for vengeance, and, what is more, for the most malignant, underhanded vengeance she can think up. She resolves to employ her son Eros as her instrument of destruction. For her the main issue is a rivalry in beauty.

The lively, sophisticated treatment of this situation should not mislead us into seeing the episode as a genre picture. Something far deeper is involved. Aphrodite and her son Eros, whom she implores by the bond of mother love, kissing him "with parted lips . . . long and fervently," are mighty, numinous gods. With the free, utterly arbitrary will of divine potentates, for whom mortal man is the "dirty muck of earth," the Great Mother and her divine son-lover set out to punish human hybris. The tale of Psyche begins with the constellation of Greek tragedy.

The radiant, malignant beauty of this immortal pair exerts a fascination which no reader of the tale can escape. Eros—the headstrong, truly "wicked boy," whose arrows threaten even his own mother and father, Aphrodite and Zeus—is asked to destroy Psyche with the weapon of Aphrodite and Eros, with love. The princess must "be consumed with passion for the vilest of men . . . one so broken that through all the world his misery has no peer." The all-powerful goddess, the Great Mother, whose primordial image breathes an aura of witchcraft and magic, including the power to turn men into beasts, displays her deadly love magic with the glittering shamelessness of a divinely merciless and truly soulless woman. Her divine beauty, overpowering vanity, and immoderate passion ally themselves with the heedless, playfully deadly power of Eros, which hurls men into such indescribable misery. Then, after Aphrodite has expressed her desire to see this lovely, virginal flower of human womanhood consumed by desperate love for a hideous, inhuman monster, she goes "to the shore hard by, where the sea ebbs and flows, and treading with rosy feet the topmost foam of the quivering waves, plunged down to the deep's dry floor. The sea gods tarried not to do her service. It was as though she had long since commanded their presence, though in truth she had but just formed the wish." And there follows an entrancing, color-drenched picture of Aphrodite cruising the sea, surrounded by Nereids singing a part song and Tritons, one blowing softly on a conch shell, another shielding her from the sun with a silk awning, a third holding a mirror before her eyes. This is the prologue in heaven.

Meanwhile, on earth, Psyche "for all her manifest beauty, had no joy of her loveliness." Lonely, without love or husband, she began to hate the "loveliness that had charmed so many nations." And her father, imploring the oracle of Apollo to send her a husband, receives the dire answer that we know.

Here begins a deeply meaningful chapter. Though the "marriage of death" is barely intimated in the prologue to the drama, it is essential to the basic mythological situation of the tale. The procession forming for the dreadful wedding, the torches burning low, "clogged with dark soot and ash," the "strains of the flute of wedlock . . . changed to the melancholy Lydian mode"—this is the matriarchal ritual of the marriage of death preceding the lament for Adonis. It is a vestige of the ancient mythical age, rising into the late fairy-tale world of the Alexandrine Aphrodite.

The ancient, primordial motif of the bride dedicated to death, of "death and the maiden," is sounded. And here we discern a central phenomenon of feminine-matriarchal psychology.

Seen from the standpoint of the matriarchal world, every marriage is a rape of Kore, the virginal bloom, by Hades, the ravishing, earthly aspect of the hostile male. From this point of view every marriage is an exposure on the mountain's summit in mortal loneliness, and a waiting for the male monster, to whom the bride is surrendered. The veiling of the bride is always the veiling of the mystery, and marriage as the marriage of death is a central archetype of the feminine mysteries.

In the profound experience of the feminine, the marriage of doom recounted in innumerable myths and tales, the maiden sacrificed to a monster, dragon, wizard, or evil spirit, is also a *hieros gamos*. The character of rape that the event assumes for womanhood expresses the projection—typical of the matriarchal phase—of the hostile element upon the man. It is inadequate, for example, to interpret the crime of the Danaïdes, who—all but one—murdered their husbands on their wedding night, as the resistance of womanhood to marriage and the patriarchal domination of the male. Unquestionably this interpretation is right, but it applies only to the last phase of a development that reaches much farther back.

The fundamental situation of the feminine, as we have elsewhere shown, is the primordial relation of identity between daughter and mother. For this reason the approach of the male always and in every case means separation. Marriage is always a mystery, but also a mystery of death. For the male—and this is inherent in the essential opposition between the masculine and the feminine—marriage, as the matriarchate recognized, is primarily an abduction, an acquisition—a rape.

When we concern ourselves with this profound mythological and psychological stratum, we must forget cultural development and the cultural forms taken by the relationship between man and woman and go back to the primordial phenomenon of the sexual encounter between them. It is not hard to see that the significance of this encounter is and must be very different for the masculine and the feminine. What for the masculine is aggression, victory, rape, and the satisfaction of desire—we need only take a look at the animal world and have the courage to recognize this stratum for man as well—is for the feminine destiny, transformation, and the profoundest mystery of life.

It is no accident that the central symbol of maidenhood is the flower, which delights man with its natural beauty, and it is extremely significant that the consummation of marriage, the destruction of virginity, should be known as "deflowering." In his interpretation of Persephone, Kerényi[1] has pointed to the death of the maiden Kore and the fluid boundary between being and nonbeing at the gates of Hades. Our aim is to provide psychological clarification of this mythological datum. For

[1] "The Psychological Aspects of the Kore," in Jung and Kerényi, *Essays on a Science of Mythology*. [See List of Works Cited.]

the feminine, the act of defloration represents a truly mysterious bond between end and beginning, between ceasing to be and entering upon real life. To experience maidenhood, womanhood, and nascent motherhood in one, and in this transformation to plumb the depths of her own existence: this is given only to the woman, and only as long as it remains open to the archetypal background of life. For good reason this act originally struck the masculine as numinous and utterly mysterious. In many places and at all times it has accordingly been abstracted from the context of private life and enacted as a rite.

It becomes particularly clear how decisive the transition from maiden-flower to fruit-mother must be in the life of the feminine, when we consider how quickly women age under primitive conditions, how quickly the strength of the fertile mother is consumed by hard work. The transition from girlhood to womanhood is always felt more keenly where, as so frequently happens, a carefree youth is immediately followed by the constraint and regularity of adulthood and marriage.

Here it may be argued that in primitive society there is often no question of a defloration, since an uninhibited and unaccented sexuality enters into the games of childhood, and that consequently the emphasis we seem to be putting on the factor of "marriage" is very much exaggerated if not entirely out of place. But as we have already pointed out, when we speak of "marriage," we have in mind an archetype or archetypal experience, and not a merely physiological occurrence. The experience of the original situation of the marriage of death may coincide with the first real consummation of marriage, the defloration, but it need not, any more than the original situation of childbearing need coincide with actual childbearing. It is true that innumerable women consummate marriage or perform the act of childbearing without going through the corresponding "experience"—as, to our surprise, we often observe in modern women—but this does not do away with the marriage situation as an archetype and central figure of feminine psychic reality. Myth is always the unconscious representation of such crucial life situations, and one of the reasons why myths are so significant for us is that we can read the true experiences of mankind in these confessions unobscured by consciousness.

Poetry, which in its highest form is animated by the same primordial images as myth, may disclose motifs and formulations which recapitulate mythical ones, and our mythological interpretation is gratifyingly confirmed when a poem strikes the same primordial note as resounds in the myth. Just this occurs in Rilke's poem "Alcestis," in which the poet, delving down far deeper than the motif of conjugal love, reaches the primordial stratum of the marriage of death.

According to the familiar tale, the gods granted Admetus the privilege of buying off his own death with the death of another. When the hour of his death had come, his mother, father, and friend were unwilling to give their life for his, but his wife Alcestis, whom Homer calls "divine among women," this wife celebrated for her conjugal love, willingly took death upon herself. Like the Egyptian Isis mourning for Osiris, the classical

Alcestis of patriarchal Greece was the "good wife," and her death, which casts a none too favorable light on her patriarchal husband, who exacted and accepted this death, becomes intelligible only when we consider that even Euripides regarded the life of a man as infinitely more valuable than that of a woman.[2]

But in Rilke's poem something different happens, simply because the poet's mythological intuition shifts the episode to the wedding day.

> *. . . and what came forth was she,*
> *a little smaller now than he had thought her,*
> *slender and sad in her pale bridal gown.*
> *The others all are but a lane for her,*
> *through which she comes and comes—(soon she'll*
> * be there,*
> *held in his arms, flung open wide in grief).*
> *Yet as he waits, she speaks; not to Admetus,*
> *but to the god who listens to her words;*
> *the others hear them only in the god.*

> *"None can replace him; none but I.*
> *I am his forfeit. For none is at an end*
> *as I am here. What am I now of that*
> *which once I was? Nothing, unless I die.*
> *Did she not tell you when she charged you then—*
> *the bridal bed that waits for us within*
> *is of the underworld? I have said farewell,*
> *farewell upon farewell.*
> *No dying soul could bid more sure farewells.*
> *I wedded*

[2] Rose, *A Handbook of Greek Mythology*, p. 141.

that all that buried lies under my husband
should flow, distill, resolve.—
Lead me away, for I will die for him."[3]

At first Rilke's interpretation might seem to be arbitrary poetic license, but when we consider it more closely we find that here again poetry has profound laws and sensuous roots, that its freedom is far from arbitrary. Modern scholarship has established that Alcestis had a number of cults and was originally a goddess.[4] The complete harmony between the modern poem and the bride-of-death motif in the myth becomes apparent when we learn that this goddess Alcestis was a Kore-Persephone, a goddess of death and the underworld, whose husband Admetus was originally the indomitable Hades himself,[5] and that she belonged to the group of the great matriarchal Pheraia goddesses who reigned in the primordial age of Greece. It was only in the course of historical development that the goddess Alcestis became the "heroine" and her divine husband the mortal king Admetus, a typical example of secondary personalization in which originally archetypal elements are reduced to a personal level.

Rilke doubtless came to know the myth in this personalized form. But what did he do, or rather, what happened to him? For him Alcestis was transformed into a bride. Moreover, she became the bride of death, Kore-Persephone, and the drama that was enacted within her transcended the personal sphere, transcended her hus-

[3] Tr. Emily Chisholm (unpublished).
[4] Philippson, *Thessalische Mythologie*, p. 88.
[5] Ibid., p. 85.

band, King Admetus. It became a dialogue between her and the god—the god of death, that is to say, the Admetus of the underworld, her original husband. The mythological constellation, overlaid by the changing times, is recaptured in poetry. The image in the poet's soul shakes off the disguise imposed on it by time and human history and emerges again in its original form from the primordial font of myth.

In his lines on Eurydice, Rilke sounds the motif of death and the maiden in still another key. Eurydice comes from death; Orpheus seeks to regain her for the upper world and life, but in her authentic being, her maidenhood, her "budlikeness," as Kerényi has said, hence in her inviolable "inherselfness," she already belongs to the perfection of death.

Hidden in herself she went. And her being dead
Fulfilled her even to fullness.
Full as a fruit with sweetness and with darkness
Was she with her great death, which was so new
That for the time she comprehended nothing.

She had attained a new virginity
And was intangible; her sex had closed
As a young flower closes towards evening,
And her pale hands were from the rites of marriage
So far estranged that even the slim god's
Endlessly gentle contact as he led her
Repelled her as a too great intimacy.[6]

Thus the archetypal efficacy of the maiden's marriage

[6] "Orpheus. Eurydice. Hermes" (tr. Leishman, p. 43).

of death extends from matriarchal prehistory, through the ritual sacrifice of the maiden and the ritual consummation of marriage, into modern times. And the marriage of death also occupies a central position in the tale of Psyche, although it seems at first to be represented merely as Aphrodite's vengeance.

Strangely enough, and incomprehensibly if we consider only Psyche's "simple-mindedness," her reply to her sentence, springing from her unconscious, is in profound accord with the mystery of the feminine faced with this situation of death. She does not respond with struggle, protest, defiance, resistance, as a masculine ego must have done in a similar situation, but, quite the contrary, with acceptance of her fate. With absolute clairvoyance she perceives the underlying meaning of what is happening, and this is the only instance in the tale where it is suggested that this meaning is known to the human characters. She replies: "When nations and peoples gave me divine honor, when with one voice they hailed me as a new Aphrodite, then was the time for you to grieve, to weep and mourn me as one dead." Taking the hybris (of mankind, of course, and not of her person, her ego) and its punishment quite for granted, she declares her readiness to be sacrificed: "I hasten to meet that blest union, I hasten to behold the noble husband that awaits me. Why do I put off and shun his coming? Was he not born to destroy all the world?" And with this, Psyche, abandoned on a lonely crag, is all at once removed from the sphere of the lamenting throng and of her parents as well.

Then comes the reversal, the surprise, the episode

which at first sight gives the strongest impression of a fairy tale. This is the third phase: Psyche in the paradise of Eros.

The marriage, ushered in with the great mythical splendor of a marriage of death, is consummated in a setting familiar to us from the much later tales of the *Arabian Nights*. There is an almost rococo lightness about the scene. "Now when night was well advanced a soft sound came to her ears. She trembled for her honor, seeing that she was all alone; she shook for terror and her fear of the unknown surpassed by far the fear of any peril that ever she had conceived. At length her unknown husband came and climbed the couch, made Psyche his bride, and departed in haste before the dawn."

Soon "what seemed strange at first by force of continued habit became a delight, and the sound of the voices cheered her loneliness and perplexity." Shortly thereafter she declares: "Sooner would I die a hundred deaths than be robbed of your sweet love. For whoever you are, I love you and adore you passionately. I love you as I love life itself. Compared with you Eros' own self would be as nothing." Yet this ecstasy in which she murmurs "Husband, sweet as honey" and "Psyche's life and love" is an ecstasy of darkness. It is a state of not-knowing and not-seeing, for her lover can only be felt and heard, but Psyche is satisfied, or so it seems, and lives in paradisaical bliss.

But every paradise has its serpent, and Psyche's nocturnal rapture cannot last forever. The intruder, the snake (of this paradise), is represented by Psyche's sisters, whose irruption brings the catastrophe, which here again is expulsion from paradise. Here we should seem to have the simple and familiar fairy-tale motif of the envious sisters. But analysis shows that fairy-tale motifs are anything but simple, that they actually consist of many different layers and are extremely meaningful.

Despite the urgent warning of Eros, Psyche meets her sisters; smitten with envy, they plot to destroy her happiness. The method they choose is again consonant with a universal motif, for the essential is not the murder of Psyche's husband, but that Psyche should be persuaded to break the taboo, to throw light on the hidden secret: in this case, to look upon her husband. For this is the prohibition that Psyche's unseen husband had imposed on her; she may not see him, she may not know "who he is." It is the ever-recurring "Never question me," the order not to enter the "closed room," whose infringement is to encompass Psyche's ruin.

How are these sisters characterized, and what is their meaning in the development of Psyche's story? Let us set aside the superficial, personal, fairy-tale traits, and seek to discern their underlying content.

Supposedly the sisters are happily married, but actually they hate their husbands to the bottom of their souls, in so far as we may speak of a soul in connection with such furies; they are prepared to leave them at once and under any conditions. Their marriages are a symbol of patriarchal slavery, typical examples of what we call "the slavery of the feminine in the patriarchate." They are "given to alien kings to be their handmaidens"; one describes her husband as older than her father, "balder than a pumpkin and feebler than any child." Thus she must play the role of a daughter to him in every respect, while her sister has the no less unpleasant life of a sick-nurse. Both sisters are intense man-haters and represent, as we may say by way of anticipation, a typical position of the matriarchate.

This contention is not hard to document. We must not take the obvious motif of envy as the ultimate attribute of the sisters, although it has its place in the total situation. The clearest symptom of the sisters' man-hating matriarchal attitude is their characterization of Psyche's husband.

When the sisters speak of the "embraces of a foul and venomous snake," when they say that the beast will devour Psyche and her child—for Psyche has meanwhile become pregnant—they are expressing more than the sexual envy of unsatisfied women. Their slander—for they speak the truth on a note of slanderous misunderstanding—springs from the sexual disgust of a violated and insulted matriarchal psyche. The sisters succeed in evoking this man-hating matriarchal stratum in Psyche herself. She finds herself in a conflict that is expressed in these simple words: "In the same body she hated the beast and loved the husband." This already transparent relation to the matriarchate and the man-slaying Danaïdes is intensified when the sisters advise Psyche not to flee from her unknown husband, but to kill him and cut off his head with a knife, an ancient symbol of castration sublimated to the spiritual sphere. The hostile male, woman as victim of the man-beast, the man's murder and castration as matriarchal symbols of self-defense or domination—how do these come to Psyche, what meaning and purpose have they in the myth of Psyche's development?

The activity of the man-hating matriarchal sisters contrasts sharply with the gentle devotion and self-effacement of Psyche, who has wholly surrendered herself to the sexual bondage—for that is what it is—of Eros. The appearance of the sisters brings the first movement into the paradise of sensual pleasure that Apuleius paints with such a wealth of color. In our interpretation the sister figures represent projections of the suppressed or totally unconscious matriarchal tendencies of Psyche herself, whose irruption produces a conflict within her. Psychologically speaking, the sisters are Psyche's "shadow" aspect, but their plurality shows that they reach down into transpersonal strata.

The appearance of the sisters for the first time gives Psyche a certain independence. Suddenly she sees her existence with Eros as a "luxurious prison" and yearns for human companionship. Thus far she has drifted along in the stream of an unconscious ecstasy, but now she sees the ghostlike unreality of her sensual paradise, and begins, in contact with her lover, to take cognizance of her womanhood. She makes "scenes" and ensnares the ensnarer with "passionate murmurs."

We must wholly disregard the surface intrigue if we wish to understand the real function and meaning of this irruption of the shadow-sisters. Paradoxical as it may seem, the sisters represent an aspect of the feminine consciousness that determines Psyche's whole subsequent development, and without which she would not be what she is, namely the feminine psyche. Despite its negative form, the anti-masculine and murderous agitation of the sisters embodies a true resistance of the feminine nature against Psyche's situation and attitude, the beginning of a higher feminine consciousness. Not that the sisters represent this consciousness, they are only its shadowy, that is, negative, precursor. But if Psyche succeeds in attaining this higher level, it is only because she starts by subordinating herself to the negative directive of her sisters. It is only by breaking the taboo that Eros has imposed on her, by responding to the seduction of her sisters, that she comes into conflict with Eros, who, as we shall show, is the foundation of her own development. As in the Biblical episode, the heeding of the serpent leads to expulsion from paradise and to a higher consciousness.

For with all its rapture is this existence in the sensual paradise of Eros not an unworthy existence? Is it not a state of blind, though impassioned, servitude, against which a feminine self-consciousness—and such is the matriarchal attitude of the feminine—must protest, against which it must raise all the arguments that are raised by the sisters? Psyche's existence is a nonexistence, a being-in-the-dark, a rapture of sexual sensuality which may fittingly be characterized as a being devoured by a demon, a monster. Eros as an unseen fascination is everything that the oracle of Apollo, cited by the sisters, has said of him, and Psyche really is his victim.[7]

[7] Psyche's existence in the dark paradise of Eros is an interesting variant of the hero's engulfment by the whale-dragon-monster. Here the containment and captivity in the darkness are overlaid by the quality of pleasure, but this situation too is archetypal and not exceptional. The danger of engulfment is often disguised by the lure of a (regressive) paradise which,

The basic law of the matriarchate forbids individual relations with the man and acknowledges the male only as an anonymous power, representing the godhead. For Psyche this anonymity is fulfilled, but at the same time she has incurred the profound, ineradicable disgrace of succumbing to this manhood, of falling into its power. From the standpoint of the matriarchate there is only one answer to this disgrace: to kill and castrate the masculine, and that is what the sisters demand of Psyche. But they not only embody regression; a higher feminine principle is also at work, as is made plain by the symbolism with which the myth literally "illuminates" Psyche's unconscious situation.

In her conflict with Eros, Psyche repeatedly resists his injunction to break off relations with her sisters; and with a puzzling persistence that appears to contradict her seeming softness, she preserves her bond with them in the face of the most urgent warning. In the course of this conflict she utters the revealing words that are the key to her inner situation: "I seek no more to see your

---

like the gingerbread house in the tale of Hansel and Gretel, conceals a devouring monster; here the devourer is the dragon Eros; in the fairy tale it is the witch. As in the night sea voyage the male solar hero kindles the light in the belly of the monster and then cuts himself out of the darkness, Psyche too, in her liberation from the prison of darkness, is equipped with light and knife. But in the masculine solar myth the hostile, killing action of the hero occupies the foreground; even where it is knowledge, it kills and "dismembers" its object, the dragon. In its feminine variant this need of knowing remains bound up with the greater need of loving. Even where the heroine Psyche is compelled to wound, she preserves her bond with her lover, whom she never ceases to conciliate and transform.

face; not even the dark of night can be a hindrance to my joy, for I hold you in my arms, light of my life."

But at the very moment when Psyche seems to accept the darkness, that is, the unconsciousness of her situation, and in seemingly total abandonment of her individual consciousness addresses her unknown and invisible lover as "light of my life," a feeling that has hitherto been unnoticeable breaks to the surface. She speaks negatively of the burdensome darkness and of her desire to know her lover. She exorcises her own fear of what is to come and reveals her unconscious awareness of what is happening. She was imprisoned in darkness, but now the drive toward light and knowledge has become imperious; at the same time she senses that a great menace is gathering over her head. This is what makes it so touching when she seeks to exorcise the reality of the darkness by addressing Eros as "light of my life." For though it is true in an ultimate sense that Eros is the light that shines before her, showing her the way through all her perils, this Eros who shows *her* the way is not the boyish youth who embraces her in the dark and seeks by every means at his disposal to restrain her from disturbing the paradise of their love.

Psyche—as the continuation of the story emphatically shows—is far from being merely "gentle" and "simple-hearted"; on the contrary, the attitude of the sisters, their protest and hostility, correspond to a current in Psyche herself. The matriarchal protest that surges up in her against the impossibility of the situation in which Eros holds her captive is borne in on her from outside by her sisters and impels her to action. It is this situation that makes possible the conflict in Psyche: "In the same body she hated the beast and loved the husband"; and it is this alone that enables the sisters to seduce her. Psyche does not know how Eros, her lover, really looks. Thus far the opposition, beast and lover, has been present in her unconscious but has not penetrated her consciousness. It is the sisters who make her conscious of the monster-beast aspect. Now Psyche comes into open conflict with her conscious love relation, in which Eros was only her "husband." She can no longer preserve her old unconscious state. She must see the real form of her partner, and thus the ambivalence, the opposition between a psyche that hates the beast and a psyche that loves the husband, is projected outward and leads to Psyche's act.

Armed with knife and lamp, Psyche approaches her unknown lover and in the light recognizes him as Eros. First she attempts to kill herself with the knife she had held ready for the "monster," but she fails. Next, while gazing at her lover in the light, she pricks her finger on one of his arrows; aflame with desire for him, she stoops to kiss him and a drop of scalding oil springs from the lamp, burning and wounding Eros, who awakens. Seeing that Psyche has disobeyed his command, he flies off and vanishes.

What does Psyche experience when, driven by the man-hating matriarchal powers, she approaches the bed to kill the supposed monster and beholds Eros? If we restore the mythical grandeur of the scene, which Apuleius' delicate filigree diminishes and almost distorts, we perceive a drama of great depth and power, a psychic transformation of unique meaning. It is the awakening of

Psyche as the psyche, the fateful moment in the life of the feminine, in which for the first time woman emerges from the darkness of her unconscious and the harshness of her matriarchal captivity and, in individual encounter with the masculine, loves, that is, recognizes, Eros. This love of Psyche's is of a very special kind, and it is only if we grasp what is new in this love situation that we can understand what it means for the development of the feminine as represented by Psyche.

The Psyche who approaches the bed on which Eros is lying is no longer the languorously ensnared being, bewitched by her senses, who lived in the dark paradise of sexuality and lust. Awakened by the incursion of her sisters, conscious of the danger that threatens her, she assumes the cruel militancy of the matriarchate as she approaches the bed to kill the monster, the male beast who has torn her from the upper world in a marriage of death and carried her off into darkness. But in the glow of the newly kindled light, with which she illumines the unconscious darkness of her previous existence, she recognizes Eros. *She loves.* In the light of her new consciousness she experiences a fateful transformation, in which she discovers that the separation between beast and husband is not valid. As the lightning bolt of love strikes her, she turns the knife against her own heart or (in other terms) wounds herself on Eros' arrow. With this she departs from the childlike, unconscious aspect of her reality and the matriarchal, man-hating aspect as well. Only in a squalid, lightless existence can Psyche mistake her lover for a beast, a violator, a dragon, and only as a childishly ignorant girl (but this too is a dark aspect) can she suppose that she is in love with a "higher husband" distinct from the lower dragon. In the light of irrupting love Psyche recognizes Eros as a god, who is the upper and the lower in one, and who connects the two.

Psyche pricks herself on Eros' arrow and bleeds. "So all unwitting, yet of her own doing, Psyche fell in love with Love." The beginning of her love was a marriage of death as dying, being-raped, and being-taken; what Psyche now experiences may be said to be a second defloration, the real, active, voluntary defloration, which she accomplishes in herself. She is no longer a victim, but an actively loving woman. She is in love, enraptured by Eros, who has seized her as a power from within, no longer as a man from without. For Eros as a man outside sleeps and knows nothing of what Psyche does and what goes on within her. And here the narrative begins to disclose a psychological acuteness that has no equal.

Psyche's act of love, in which she voluntarily gives herself to love, to Eros, is at once a sacrifice and a loss. She does not renounce the matriarchal stage of her womanhood; the paradoxical core of the situation is that in and through her act of love she raises the matriarchal stage to its authentic being and exalts it to the Amazonian level.

The knowing Psyche, who sees Eros in the full light and has broken the taboo of his invisibility, is no longer naïve and infantile in her attitude toward the masculine; she is no longer merely captivating and captivated, but is so completely changed in her new womanhood that she loses and indeed must lose her lover. In this love situation of womanhood growing conscious through encounter, knowledge and suffering and sacrifice are identical. With Psyche's love that burst forth when she "sees Eros," there comes into being within her an Eros who is no longer identical with the sleeping Eros outside her. This inner Eros that is the image of her love is in truth a higher and invisible form of the Eros who lies sleeping before her. It is the adult Eros which pertains to the conscious, adult psyche, the Psyche who is no longer a child. This greater, invisible Eros within Psyche must necessarily come into conflict with his small, visible incarnation who is revealed by the light of her lamp and burned by the drop of oil. The Eros hidden in the darkness could still be an embodiment of every image of Eros that lived within Psyche, but the Eros who has become visible is the divine, finite reality of the boy who is Aphrodite's son.[8]

And, we must not forget, Eros himself did *not* want such a Psyche! He threatened her, he fervently implored her to remain in the paradise-darkness, he warned her that she would lose him forever by her act. The unconscious tendency toward consciousness (here toward consciousness in the love relationship) was stronger in Psyche than everything else, even than her love for Eros—or so, at least, the masculine Eros would have said. But wrongly

[8] But for Psyche it is essential that she unify the dual structure of Eros, which is also manifested in the antithetical figures of Eros and Anteros, and transform the lower into the higher Eros. Here it is interesting to note that the twofold Eros, the Eros of Aphrodite and the Eros of Psyche, "τῆς Ἀφροδίτης καὶ τῆς ψυχῆς Ἔρωτα," is already mentioned in the Egyptian magic papyrus. See Reitzenstein, *Das Märchen von Amor und Psyche bei Apuleius*, p. 80.

so, for though the Psyche of the paradisaical state was subservient to Eros, though she had yielded to him in the darkness, she had not loved him. Something in her, which may be designated negatively as matriarchal aggression, or positively as a tendency toward consciousness and a fulfillment precisely of her feminine nature, drove her imperiously to emerge from the darkness. It is in the light of knowledge, her knowledge of Eros, that she begins to love.

The loss of her lover in this moment is among the deepest truths of this myth; this is the tragic moment in which every feminine psyche enters upon its own destiny. Eros is wounded by Psyche's act; the drop of oil that burns him, awakens him, and drives him away is in every sense a source of pain. To him, the masculine god, she was desirable enough when she was in the dark and he possessed her in the dark, when she was the mere companion of his nights, secluded from the world, living only for him, without share in his diurnal existence, in his reality and his divinity. Her servitude was made still deeper by his insistence on his divine anonymity: she was still more "devoured" by him. This childlike girl, this "simple and gentle soul" (a masculine misunderstanding if ever there was one!), approaches the sleeper with knife and lamp to slay him. Inevitably her willingness to lose him must burn and wound the masculine Eros most painfully.

Psyche emerges from the darkness and enters upon her destiny as a woman in love, for she is Psyche, that is, her essence is psychic, an existence in paradisaical darkness cannot satisfy her.[9] It is not until Psyche experiences Eros as more than the darkly ensnaring one, not until she sees him (*he* after all has always seen her), that she really encounters him. And in this very moment of loss and alienation, she loves him and consciously recognizes Eros.

With this she enacts the matriarchal sacrifice of the lover on a higher plane and with the full justification of her human claim to consciousness. By freeing herself from him with dagger and lamp, which she bears in place of the torch of Hecate and the other matriarchal goddesses, and so surpassing him and her servitude to him, she deprives Eros of his divine power over her. Psyche and Eros now confront one another as equals. But confrontation implies separateness. The uroboric[10] original unity of the embrace in the darkness is transcended, and with Psyche's heroic act suffering, guilt, and loneliness have come into the world. For Psyche's act is analogous to the deed of the hero who separated the original parents in order to produce the light of consciousness; in this case, it is Psyche and Eros themselves, during their sojourn in the paradise of darkness, who are the original parents.

But Psyche's act only appears to be a "masculine" deed

---

[9] This is a repetition on a different plane of the matriarchal act of the Amazon, who sacrifices her womanhood, her breasts, not only in order to fight as a man in her struggle with the male for independence, but also in order to fortify the Great Goddess of the matriarchate. The "many-breasted" Ephesian Artemis wears a cloak of breasts, which are the symbols of the breasts sacrificed to her by the Amazons, if not these breasts themselves. Cf. Picard, "Die Ephesia von Anatolien," *EJ 1938*.

[10] The uroboros is the circular snake, biting its tail, that symbolizes the One and All.

resembling that of the hero. For there is one crucially and fundamentally different factor: although Psyche's act corresponds to the necessary development of consciousness, it is not an act of killing, indeed it is this very act that gives rise to Psyche's love. And whereas the masculine goes on from his act of heroic slaying to conquer the world, whereas his *hieros gamos* with the anima figure he has won constitutes only a part of his victory,[11] Psyche's subsequent development is nothing other than an attempt to transcend, through suffering and struggle, the separation accomplished by her act. On a new plane, that is, in love and full consciousness, she strives to be reunited with him who had been separated from her and make whole again by a new union what necessity had impelled her to sacrifice. Thus Psyche's act is the beginning of a development which not only embraces Psyche but must also seize hold of Eros.

Eros, as he himself relates, was wounded at the very outset by his own arrow, that is, he loved Psyche from the start, whereas Psyche, who wounds herself in accomplishing her deed, falls in love with Eros only in this moment. But what Eros calls "his love" and the manner in which he wishes to love her conflict with Psyche and her act. By her courageous readiness to embark on her independent development, to sacrifice him in order to know him, Psyche drives Eros and herself out of the paradise of uroboric unconsciousness. It is through Psyche's act that Eros first suffers the consequence of the arrow of love that he has aimed at himself.[12]

[11] Cf. my *Origins and History of Consciousness*, pp. 195 ff.

[12] It need not concern us that this is a logical development of the mythical figure of Eros, who was originally less and more than an actual god.

Here something should be said about the symbolism of the scalding oil that burns Eros. "Ah! rash, overbold lamp!" says our tale, "thou burnest the very lord of fire." The bringer of suffering is not a cutting weapon, like the arrow, but the substance that feeds the lamp, which is the principle of light and knowledge. The oil as essence of the plant world, an essence of the earth, which is accordingly used to anoint the lord of the earth, the king, is a widespread symbol. In this case it is significant as the basis of light, and to give light it must kindle and burn. Similarly in psychic life, it is the heat, the fire of passion, the flame and ardor of emotion that provide the basis of illumination, that is, of an illumined consciousness, which rises from the combustion of the fundamental substance and enhances it.

Through her act Psyche achieves consciousness of Eros and her love, but Eros is only wounded and is by no means illumined by Psyche's act of love and separation. In him only one part of the necessary process is fulfilled: the basic substance is kindled, and he is burned by it. He is stricken with an affective pain, and through Psyche's act he is flung from the intoxication of blissful union into the pain of suffering. But the transformation is involuntary, and he experiences it passively.

When gods love mortals, they experience only desire and pleasure. The suffering had always been left to the mortal part, the human, who was usually destroyed by the encounter, while the divine partner went smilingly on to new adventures equally disastrous for humankind. But here something different happens: Psyche, for all her individuality a symbol of mortal woman's soul, takes an active part.

Eros, as we have seen in the beginning, was a boy, a youth, the son-lover of his great mother. He has circumvented Aphrodite's commandment and loved Psyche instead of making her unhappy—but has he really circumvented her command, has he not made her unhappy after all, has he not forced her into marriage with a monster, the "vilest of men"? In any event, he has not freed himself from the Mother Goddess but has merely deceived her behind her back. For his design was that everything should take place in darkness and secrecy, hidden from the eyes of the goddess. His "affair" with Psyche was planned as one of the many little digressions of Greek gods, far from the light of public opinion, which is typically represented by the feminine deities.

This situation with all its advantages for Eros is disturbed by Psyche. Psyche dissolves her *participation mystique* with her partner and flings herself and him into the destiny of separation that is consciousness. Love as an expression of feminine wholeness is not possible in the dark, as a merely unconscious process; an authentic encounter with another involves consciousness, hence also the aspect of suffering and separation.

Psyche's act leads, then, to all the pain of individuation, in which a personality experiences itself in relation to a partner as something other, that is, as not only connected with the partner. Psyche wounds herself and wounds Eros, and through their related wounds their original, unconscious bond is dissolved. But it is this two-fold wounding that first gives rise to love, whose striv-

ing it is to reunite what has been separated; it is this
wounding that creates the possibility of an encounter,
which is prerequisite for love between two individuals.
In Plato's *Symposium* the division of the One and the
yearning to reunite what has been sundered are represented as the mythical origin of love; here this same insight is repeated in terms of the individual.

Bachofen writes: "The power that leads back together
again that which has been cut apart is the egg-born god,
whom the Orphic teachings call Metis, Phanes, Erico-
paeus, Protogonos, Heracles, Thronos, Eros, the Lesbians
Enorides, the Egyptians Osiris."[18] There the feminine is
always the egg and the container, while the masculine is
that which is born and that which parts the primordial
unity; in our context, however, the exact opposite is true.
Eros, the Eros of Aphrodite, holds Psyche captive, ensnared in the darkness of the egg, and Psyche, with knife
and lamp, parts this perfect existence of the beginning;
with her acts and sufferings she restores the original
unity on a celestial plane.

Psyche's act ends the mythical age in the archetypal
world, the age in which the relation between the sexes
depended only on the superior power of the gods, who
held men at their mercy. Now begins the age of human
love, in which the human psyche consciously takes the
fateful decision on itself. And this brings us to the background of our myth, namely the conflict between Psyche,
the "new Aphrodite," and Aphrodite as the Great
Mother.

[18] Bachofen, *Versuch über die Gräbersymbolik der Alten*, pp.
93 ff.

The rivalry began when men, beholding the beauty of Psyche, neglected the cult and the temples of Aphrodite. This pure contemplation of beauty is in itself contrary to the principle represented by Aphrodite. Aphrodite, too, is beautiful and represents beauty, but her beauty is only a means to an end. The end seems to be desire and sexual intoxication; actually it is fertility. Aphrodite is the Great Mother, the "original source of all five elements." When, like the Babylonian Ishtar and the Greek Demeter, she hides herself in anger, the world grows barren. "After the Lady Ishtar has descended, the bull no longer mounts the cow, the ass no longer bends over the she-ass, and the man no longer bends over the woman in the street: the man slept in his place, the woman slept alone."[14]

When Kerényi says: "Aphrodite is no more a fertility goddess than is Demeter or Hera,"[15] he negatively establishes the term "fertility goddess" in order to reject it. But all three, as "primal source of all the elements," are manifestations of the Great Mother, the matriarchal creatrix of life and of the fertility of living things; and it is this aspect, and this alone, that gave the Great Mother her original dignity, the queenship by virtue of which she invested the king with his power. Hence, although Aphrodite as goddess represents an eternal sphere of being, she is only one aspect of the archetype of the Great Mother. Aphrodite's beauty, seductiveness, and pleasure giving are weapons in a celestial sport, like the color of

[14] "Die Höllenfahrt der Ischtar," in Ungnad, *Die Religion der Babylonier und Assyrier.*

[15] Kerényi, *Töchter der Sonne*, p. 165.

the flower, which, reaching beyond its beauty and charm, serves the primordial-maternal purpose of the species.

But the alliance represented by Aphrodite and Eros also embraces the beauty and charm of human relations, as is revealed by the words of the sea mew, who declares that the world is out of sorts because Eros has flown down to some mountain "to revel with a harlot" and that Aphrodite herself has abandoned her divine tasks and gone off for a seaside holiday. "And so there has been no pleasure, no joy, no merriment anywhere, but all things lie in rude unkempt neglect; wedlock and true friendship and parents' love for their children have vanished from the earth; there is one vast disorder, one hateful loathing and foul disregard of all bonds of love."

When Aphrodite vents her indignation over Eros' love, Hera and Demeter speak even more plainly: "Who among gods and men will permit you to sow passions broadcast among the peoples of the earth, while you forbid your own household the charms of love, and debar them from all enjoyment of woman's foibles, an enjoyment that is open to all the world?" The sowing of "passions" and rule over "woman's foibles" are Aphrodisian attributes of the Great Mother, and in what high degree the "old" Aphrodite still represents this aspect is evident from her conflict with Psyche.

Aphrodite's indignation begins when, in the human realm, whose nature it was to serve her, to celebrate her power, and to do her work—when in this realm of "earthly muck" something absurd happens, when the "new Aphrodite" is worshiped in pure contemplation. Helen was still Aphrodite's true handmaiden, for she aroused desire and fomented war, the fateful movement of human heroism which Aphrodite loved in Mars. For the phallic power of Mars is connected with blood lust, which had always been closely related to sexual lust. Helen, like Aphrodite, never ceased to renew the calamitous mixtures of rapture, magic, and destruction that make up the fascination of the Great Mother, who is also a mother of fate and death. But what is Psyche, this "new Aphrodite," who is beautiful, yet not desired by humankind, but instead, though human, is worshiped contemplatively like a goddess, and, worst of all, desired by the divine Eros?

Psyche intervenes in the sphere of the gods and creates a new world. With her act the feminine as a human psychic force comes into conflict with the Great Mother and her terrible aspect, to which the matriarchal existence of the feminine had been subservient. And Psyche turns not only against the Great Mother, against Aphrodite, the mighty ruler over feminine existence, but also against her masculine lover, against Eros. How feeble is the position of the human Psyche in this struggle with the gods and powers! How hopeless seems her situation, the situation of the feminine-human life principle that dares to set itself against a divine archetype!

With the self-sacrifice of her act she gives up everything and enters into the loneliness of a love in which, at once unconsciously and consciously, she renounces the attraction of her beauty that leads to sex and fertility. Once she sees Eros in the light, Psyche sets the love principle of encounter and individuation beside the principle of fascinating attraction and the fertility of the species.

In this context we can understand the mythological "genealogies" according to which Aphrodite is born of union between the generative sky and the sea, while Psyche, the "new Aphrodite," is the product of a union of heaven and earth. For the sea preserves all the anonymity that is characteristic of the collective unconscious, while the earth symbolizes the higher, "earthly" form. Aphrodite represents the union of the anonymous powers of Above and Below; in uniting the masculine and feminine she operates as a universal and anonymous power. With Psyche, an earthly, human realization of the same Aphrodisian principle has come into being on a higher plane. But earthly and human means unique, in accord with the principle of individuality and—ultimately—of individuation. Over the material-psychic love principle of Aphrodite as goddess of the mutual attraction between opposites rises Psyche's love principle, which with this attraction connects knowledge, the growth of consciousness, and psychic development. With Psyche, then, there appears a new love principle, in which the encounter between feminine and masculine is revealed as the basis of individuation. From the standpoint of Aphrodite as a nature principle, the union of feminine with masculine is not essentially different in man and in the animals, from the snakes and wolves to the doves. But once the relation between Psyche and Eros has transcended this stage through Psyche's act, it represents a psychology of encounter; a uniquely loving one fulfills his existence through this love, which embraces suffering and separation.

For the first time Psyche's individual love rises up in

mythological rebellion against the collective principle of sensual drunkenness represented by Aphrodite. Paradoxical as it may sound, poor Psyche has still to conquer, in fact to develop, her lover. Aphrodite's son-beloved must become a human lover, Eros must be saved from the transpersonal sphere of the Great Mother and brought into the personal sphere of the human Psyche. It remains to be seen whether Psyche will prove stronger than Aphrodite, whether she will succeed in winning Eros.

In this situation Aphrodite regresses into the wicked mother, the stepmother and witch of the fairy tales. "You trample your mother's bidding underfoot," she screams at Eros, "instead of tormenting my enemy with base desires!" She behaves like a "terrible mother," as grotesque as any we find described in the textbooks of psychology. She sounds the motif of the outraged mother who fears that a daughter-in-law will carry off her son, hitherto held captive in an incestuous relationship, and rings all the changes on it. "Matricidal wretch!" she calls Eros at the height of her harangue, and here we must recall that when she first set out to ruin Psyche, she had implored this son "by all the bonds of love that bind us" and "with parted lips kissed her son long and fervently." And of course she points out that this son owes everything to her and her alone and swears to acquire another son. How very earthly and familiar it sounds to the psychologist when she cries: "Truly, I am highly blessed that I should be called a grandmother, though yet in the flower of my age, and that the son of a vile serving-wench should be known as Aphrodite's grandchild!"

But why, one may reasonably ask, does Aphrodite regress into the Bad Mother rather than the Great Mother; why do all the personalistic traits of family life come out in her, rather than the mythological traits of the Great Mother, as we might expect?

Throughout this tale the principle of "secondary personalization"[16] is dominant. With developing consciousness, transpersonal and archetypal phenomena have assumed a personal form and taken their place in the framework of an individual history, a human life situation. The human psyche is an active ego which dares to oppose transpersonal forces—and successfully so. The consequence of this enhanced position of the human, here the feminine, personality is to enfeeble what was formerly all-powerful. The tale of Psyche ends with the deification of the human Psyche. Correspondingly, the divine Aphrodite becomes human, and so likewise Eros, who through suffering prepares the way for union with the human Psyche.

When it becomes clear to Aphrodite that her masculine offspring, who has always been her obedient slave, has exceeded his function of son-beloved, instrument and helper, and made himself independent as a lover, a conflict arises within the feminine sphere, and a new phase begins in the development of Eros. Psyche, the human woman, sets herself up against the Great Mother, who hitherto, in league with her son, had prescribed the destinies of human love. In establishing an independent feminine consciousness of love through free encounter, Psyche rejects the dark anonymous love that consisted only

[16] My *Origins*, index, s.v.

of drunken lust and fertility, the transpersonal love that had hitherto governed all life. And in rejecting Aphrodite she also rejects an Eros who fears Aphrodite's authority and at most circumvents her in secret, but does not dare to stand independently by the side of his loved one. In rejecting both Aphrodite and Eros, Psyche, all unknowing and unwilling, enters into a heroic struggle of the feminine that ushers in a new human era.

In her wrath Aphrodite turns to Demeter and Hera, who grant their support neither to her nor to Psyche when she appeals to them for help. They remain neutral in the conflict that has broken out in the realm of the feminine, to which they too belong. Fundamentally they belong to Aphrodite, their threefold power is opposed to Psyche, but fear of Eros holds them in check.

When Psyche abandons her flight from Aphrodite, which is really a quest for Eros, and surrenders to the goddess, she is prepared for "certain death."

Aphrodite's plan to destroy Psyche revolves around the four labors that she imposes upon her. In performing these four strange and difficult labors in the service of Aphrodite, Psyche becomes a feminine Heracles; her mother-in-law plays the same role as Heracles' stepmother. In both cases the Bad Mother plays the role of destiny, and in both cases this destiny leads to heroism and "memorable deeds." For us the essential is to note how the heroism of the feminine differs from that of the masculine.

The labors imposed on Psyche by Aphrodite seem at first sight to present neither meaning nor order. But an interpretation based on an understanding of the symbolism of the unconscious shows the exact opposite to be true.[17]

The first labor, to sort out a huge mound of barley, millet, poppy seed, peas, lentils, and beans, is known to us from the tale of Cinderella and many other fairy tales.[18] Aphrodite introduces it with the cynical words: "I cannot conceive that any serving-wench as hideous as yourself could find any means to attract lovers save by making herself their drudge; wherefore now I myself will make trial of your worth." Here Aphrodite sounds like a fishwife, and a particularly coarse and mean one at that. We mention this not for the sake of moral indignation, but because these touches in the narrative disclose the depths of the conflict. What interests us is not the characterization of Aphrodite's nastiness, but the hatred of a goddess and queen menaced in the very core of her being.

Obviously Aphrodite thinks that this first labor is impossible to perform. It consists in sorting out a hopeless muddle of seeds. The mound of seeds primarily sym-

[17] Our interpretation of Psyche's labors is the product of a collective effort. It grew out of a seminar in Tel-Aviv, in which the author expounded his "psychology of the feminine," of which the chapter on Psyche forms a part. Valuable additions were also made by the members of a course on the tale of Psyche at the C. G. Jung Institute, in Zurich.

Here I should like to thank the members of these seminars, whose collaboration made it possible for me to interpret this section of the tale, which at first struck me as incoherent. I wish also to thank Dr. Jung and Mrs. Jung for their useful comments on my manuscript.

[18] Weinreich, "Das Märchen von Amor und Psyche," ch. x in Friedländer, *Darstellungen aus der Sittengeschichte Roms*, Vol. IV.

bolizes a uroboric mixture of the masculine, that is to say, a promiscuity typical of Bachofen's swamp stage.[19] The creatures that come to Psyche's help are not the doves, the birds of Aphrodite, which many centuries later come to the help of Cinderella, but the ants, the myrmidons, the "nimble nurslings of earth, the mother of all."

What does it mean that Psyche, aided by the ants, should succeed in putting order into masculine promiscuity? Kerényi[20] has pointed to the primordial human character of the earthborn ant peoples and their connection with autochthony, that is, the earthborn nature of life and particularly of man.

Here, as always, the helpful animals are symbols of the instinct world. When we reflect that the ants are known to us from dreams as a symbol correlated with the "vegetative" nervous system, we begin to understand why these chthonian powers, these creatures born of the earth, are able to order the masculine seeds of the earth. Psyche counters Aphrodite's promiscuity with an instinctual ordering principle. While Aphrodite holds fast to the fertility of the swamp stage, which is also represented by Eros in the form of a dragon, a phallic serpent-monster, Psyche possesses within her an unconscious principle which enables her to select, sift, correlate, and evaluate, and so find her way amid the confusion of the masculine. In opposition to the matriarchal position of

[19] Bachofen's "hetaerism" should be understood as a psychic stratum and phase, namely the uroboric phase characterized by the relation of identity, not as a historical or social fact.

[20] "Urmensch und Mysterien," *EJ 1947.*

Aphrodite, for whom the masculine is anonymous—and fundamentally so, as is shown by the rites of Ishtar, for example, and by many mysteries—Psyche, even in her first labor, has reached the stage of selectivity. Even at this dark stage she is aided by an ordering instinct which illumines her situation with the "light of nature."

This brings us to a more universal interpretation of the labor. The confused heap of seeds, fruits, and grains also represents the disordered welter of fruitful predispositions and potentialities that are present in the feminine nature as understood by Aphrodite. Psyche's act brings order into them and so for the first time enables them to develop. An unconscious spiritual principle is already at work within Psyche. It works for her and by putting order into matter makes it serviceable to her.

In other words, Psyche's development does not run counter to the unconscious and the instincts, the "powers of the earth." She represents, to be sure, a development toward consciousness, light, and individuation, but, in contrast with the corresponding development in the male, she preserves the umbilical cord that attaches her to the unconscious foundation.[21] The "neutrality" of Hera and Demeter may also be understood in this light. The conflict between Psyche and Aphrodite takes place in the sphere of the feminine. It is not a conflict between an individual, whether man or woman, and the feminine-maternal which this individual seeks to relinquish or directly oppose. We have stressed that Psyche's behavior

[21] Characteristically, "fools" and children have a similar development in fairy tales and myth. They too are often helped by animals.

is "feminine," and the narrative contains innumerable allusions to this fact. Her naïveté, as well as the type of scene to which she subjects Eros, her "passionate murmurs," as well as her propensity for despair, are thoroughly feminine. Still more so is the quality of her love and will, which, though not unswerving as in men, are for all their suppleness amazingly tenacious and firm.

Let us not forget who it is that Psyche first meets after Eros has forsaken her and after the river has frustrated her attempt at suicide, so proving to her that regression is impossible. As so often in this tale, what would seem to be a mere incidental, a touch in an idyllic genre picture, proves to be filled with profound mythological meaning. "It chanced that at that moment Pan, the god of the countryside, sat on the river's brow with Echo, the mountain goddess, in his arms, teaching her. . . ." With his "divination," as "men that are wise call it," he recognizes her situation at once, and it is he who gives Psyche the lesson with which she goes on living, and which profoundly influences the whole ensuing action. "Address Eros, the mightiest of gods, with fervent prayer and win him by tender submission, for he is an amorous and soft-hearted youth."

Pan is the god of natural existence, taught by "long old age and ripe experience," a "rustic shepherd," close to the earth and animals, a lover of life and living creatures—hence the benefits of "long old age." His advice to Psyche is this: Eros is the greatest of the gods; and as for you, Psyche, be feminine and win his love. It is no accident that he has Echo in his arms, the unattainable beloved, who transforms herself into music for him, and with whom he holds an eternal loving dialogue. He is wise, loving, natural, Psyche's true mentor. His figure remains entirely in the background, and yet this "old sage" determines Psyche's development.

On the surface the labors that Aphrodite imposes on Psyche are only deadly perils devised by the hostile, treacherous goddess with a view to destroying her. But Pan's advice that Psyche should win Eros' love brings meaning into what seemed meaningless. It is through these words of the old sage that Aphrodite's labors become Psyche's acts. It is because Pan has opened Psyche's eyes to the meaning hidden in Aphrodite's seemingly arbitrary labors that the events take on a direction, namely a direction toward Eros, and that Psyche's course from labor to labor becomes a *way*.

The second, still stranger labor that Aphrodite demands of Psyche is to gather a hank of the wool of the "shining golden sheep." Here it is the whispering reeds that tell Psyche how to go about it. What is this labor exacted by Aphrodite? how does Psyche manage to perform it? what does it mean? and what is the role of the "kind and simple-hearted reed"?

The sheep, or rather rams, whose wool Psyche is expected to gather, are described by the reed as destructive magic powers. The reed's words make their relation to the sun clear enough, even if we did not know the solar significance of the ram from Egypt, from the legend of the Golden Fleece, and various other examples.[22]

Psyche is warned against going among these "terrible" sheep until the sun has gone down. "For they borrow

[22] Kerényi, *Töchter*, pp. 30 ff.

fierce heat from the blazing sun and wild frenzy maddens them, so that with sharp horns and foreheads hard
as stone, and sometimes even with venomous bites, they
vent their fury in the destruction of men." The rams of
the sun, symbols of the destructive power of the masculine, correspond to the negative masculine death principle as experienced by the matriarchate. Cynically con-
fident that this will be her doom, Aphrodite sends the
feminine Psyche to disarm and rob this destructive masculine principle, the devouring sun, whose hair-rays are
the wool of the solar ram. For this, as so often in myth,
is the meaning behind the order to steal a hair, a lock
of hair, and so forth. And this symbolic "castration"
must be taken to signify a taking-possession-of, an overpowering, a "depotentiation."[23] This is the meaning of
Delilah's shearing of Samson, the solar hero, and of the
primordial, Amazonian crime of the Danaïdes.

Psyche seems condemned to destruction by the overpowering masculine principle; it seems as though she
must melt in the destructive noonday fire of this masculine solar power, for the rending golden rams of the
sun symbolize an archetypally overpowering male-spirit-
ual power which the feminine cannot face. The archetypal power of this deadly spiritual principle is that of
the "paternal uroboros"[24] in its negative aspect, in contact with which the feminine must burn like Semele in
the presence of Zeus, or go mad like the daughters of
Minyas,[25] who vainly opposed Dionysus. Only a total

[23] My *Origins*, p. 59.
[24] Cf. my "Die psychologischen Stadien der weiblichen Entwicklung."
[25] Aelian, *Varia hist.*, III, 42.

religious openness toward this spiritual principle that turns its creative aspect toward the feminine can enable the feminine to survive. But then it is captivated by the masculine, with all the blessings and perils that such a seizure involves.

The rams, however, represent the negative aspect of this principle, whose deadly aggression is a symbol of the fatal incursion of the unconscious powers into the psyche. On the personal level this is manifested from the first in Psyche's tendency toward suicide. Psyche feels unequal to the struggle with the archetypal world—the nature of the gods. Over and over again it proves too much for her. It is only with increasing integration, with the advancing development of the self, that the human Psyche can resist this assault. Once again Psyche seems doomed to failure.

But she is aided by the reed, the hair of the earth, that is connected with the water of the depths, the contrary element to the ram fire—and it is from the water that the reed derives its elastic suppleness. The reed whispers to her with his Pan-like, vegetative wisdom, the wisdom of growth: wait, be patient. Things change. Time brings counsel. It is not always high noon, and the masculine is not always deadly. One must not attack with force. A time will come when the sun is no longer at the zenith but on its way to set, a time when the heat is no longer rabid and ruinous. Evening comes, and night, when the sun returns home, when the masculine principle approaches the feminine and Helios "journeys to the depths of the sacred dark night, to the mother and to his wife and many children."[26]

[26] Stesichorus, quoted in Kerényi, *Töchter*, p. 28.

Then, as the sun is setting, there arises the love situation in which it is natural and safe to take the golden hair of the sun rams. Both physically and psychically these hair-rays are the fructifying powers of the masculine, and the feminine, as positive Great Mother, is the great Weaver who plaits the threads of the sun seeds into the web of nature.[27] A parallel is the negative deed of Delilah, who steals the hair of Samson as he sleeps, exhausted by the feats of love. She too is a nocturnal feminine figure whose personalized form, like that of Samson, conceals a mythical figure.[28]

Thus the ruin of the feminine, as planned by Aphrodite, is averted with the help of the reed; the feminine need only consult its instinct in order to enter into a fruitful relation, that is to say, a love relation, with the masculine at nightfall. And thus the situation in which masculine and feminine face one another in deadly hostility is transcended.

The wisdom of the mantic reed proves superior to the keen knowledge of the burning and killing male spiritual principle. This feminine wisdom belongs to the "matriarchal consciousness,"[29] which in its waitful, vegetative, nocturnal way takes "what it needs" from the killing power of the male solar spirit. It does not expose itself to the killing fullness of the ram's power; for, if the feminine strove to take what it requires by confronting the ram directly, it would be doomed to destruction. But

[27] Ibid., p. 81.
[28] She is negatively feminine, the destructive anima; but she is also the deadly mother goddess of Canaan in struggle with the YHWH principle and with consciousness.
[29] My "Über den Mond und das matriarchale Bewusstsein."

at nightfall, when the masculine solar spirit returns to the feminine depths, the feminine—as though in passing—finds the golden strand, the fruitful seed of light.

Here again the solution to the problem consists not in struggle but in the creation of a fruitful contact between feminine and masculine. Psyche is an exact reversal of Delilah. She does not rob a disarmed and enfeebled man of his power in order to kill him in the manner of the Terrible Mother and the kindred figure of the negative anima. Nor does she, like Medea, steal the Golden Fleece by trickery and violence; she finds the element of the masculine that is necessary to her in a peaceful situation, without harming the masculine in any way.

In our interpretation, the two first labors thus present an "erotic problem." And strange to say, Aphrodite, who had presented these labors not as an "erotic problem," but as a sorting out of seeds and the quest for a strand of golden wool, attributes the solution to the help of Eros. "I am well aware who was the secret author of this deed." And yet she must have known perfectly well that Eros was sick and imprisoned in her palace. In spite of everything there seems to be some hidden rapport between Aphrodite and Psyche through which Aphrodite understands the "erotic" character not only of her problems, but also of Psyche's solutions.

On the surface, the third labor seems unrelated to this context. Aphrodite sends Psyche to fill a crystal vessel with the water of the spring that feeds Styx and Cocytus, the streams of the underworld. The undertaking seems perfectly hopeless. The spring flows from the highest crag of a huge mountain; it is guarded by eternally watchful snakes, and Psyche is further discouraged by the stream itself, which murmurs to her: "Hence! Beware!" Here the deus ex machina is Zeus' eagle, who had carried off Ganymede and who, remembering the assistance given him by Eros on this occasion, comes to Psyche's help.

This labor is a variant of the quest for the water of life, the precious substance hard to obtain. It is nowhere mentioned what qualities the water of our spring possesses, and not even implied that it is any special kind of water. Hence we may assume that the secret does not lie in the quality of the water but in the specific difficulty of attaining it. The essential feature of this spring is that it unites the highest and lowest; it is a uroboric circular stream that feeds the depths of the underworld and rises up again to issue from the highest crag of the "huge mountain." The problem is to capture in a vessel the water of this spring, symbolizing the stream of vital energy, an Oceanus or a Nile on a reduced mythical scale. Aphrodite regards the task as hopeless, because to her mind the stream of life defies capture, it is eternal movement, eternal change, generation, birth, and death. The essential quality of this stream is precisely that it cannot be contained. Psyche then, as feminine vessel, is ordered to contain the stream, to give form and rest to what is formless and flowing; as vessel of individuation, as mandala-urn, she is ordered to mark off a configured unity from the flowing energy of life, to give form to life.

Here it becomes evident that, in addition to its general meaning as the uncontainable energy of the unconscious, the life stream possesses a specific symbolism in

Creativity?

{ 103 }

relation to Psyche. As what fills the mandala-urn this stream is male-generative, like the archetypally fecundating power of innumerable river gods all over the world. In relation to the feminine psyche it is the overwhelming male-numinous power of that which penetrates to fructify, that is, of the paternal uroboros. The insoluble problem which Aphrodite sets Psyche, and which Psyche solves, is to encompass this power without being shattered by it.

For a better understanding of this context, we must interpret the various symbols that appear in the text. What does it mean that the eagle should make possible the performance of this labor? Why the eagle, this masculine spirit symbol, belonging to Zeus and the realm of the air? And why, in particular, "the eagle of Ganymede," who carried off Zeus' favorite to Olympus? Here many motifs seem to be intertwined, but all serve to clarify the situation of Psyche in her conflict with Aphrodite.

To begin with, there is an evident parallel between Ganymede and Psyche. Both are human beings loved by gods, and both are ultimately carried off to Olympus as earthly-heavenly companions of their divine lovers. This is the first intimation of Zeus' sympathy with Psyche, which decides the final outcome of her story. He sides with his son, Eros, partly out of masculine sympathy, for he too knows the meaning of seizure by love, and partly out of protest against the Great Goddess, who as Hera strives to check her husband's freedom to love, and as Aphrodite tries to restrict her son in the same way.

It is no accident that the homosexual love relation of Zeus and Ganymede should come to the help of Eros and Psyche. Elsewhere[30] we have shown that homoerotic and homosexual male pairs act as "strugglers," taking up the war of liberation against the domination of the Great Mother. And here again Eros must be freed from his status as a son-lover before he can enter into a free and independent relation with Psyche.

It is not irrelevant to what has gone before that the masculine spirit aspect, whose central symbol is the eagle, should come to Psyche's aid in this third labor. The second labor, according to our interpretation, consisted in the "taming" of the hostile masculine principle, in the erotic binding of what might have been destructive in the form of the paternal uroboros. It is this reconciliation with the masculine that enables Psyche to enter into communication with the masculine spirit world of Ganymede's eagle. In the first labor the instinctual powers of nature had worked "unconsciously," as it were, in their ordering and sifting; in the second, Psyche had managed to avoid the overpowering assault of the masculine spirit and to take from it what was necessary and fruitful for her, the single strand of golden wool. In the third labor a further development befalls her. The spiritual principle that helps her, the eagle of the masculine spirit, who spies the booty and carries it off, enables her to contain some of the living stream of life and give it form. The eagle holding the vessel profoundly symbolizes the already male-female spirituality of Psyche, who in one act "receives" like a woman, that is, gathers like a vessel and conceives, but at the same time apprehends and knows like a man. The circular power of this life stream,

[30] My *Origins*, pp. 96 f.

which is experienced by the feminine psyche as both male-fecundating and overpowering, belongs to the pre-configurative stage that we designate as paternal uroboros. Its blinding, destructive brightness is symbolized in the sun rams, while its uncontainable, overpowering energy is embodied in the circular stream. The masculine principle of the eagle enables Psyche to receive a part of it without being destroyed.

In the one instance, a strand of wool is detached from the fullness of the light; in the other, a cupful of water is removed from the fullness of the stream. Both symbols, on different planes, mean that Psyche can receive and assimilate the masculine and give it form, without being destroyed by the overwhelming power of the numinosum.

Because Psyche is born of the earth, she can only receive and give form to a part of the infinite that is within her reach, but this precisely is what befits her and makes her human. This capacity for form-giving limitation is the basis of the principle of individuation that she embodies. In designating the pile of disordered seeds in the first labor, the destructive masculine brightness of the second, and the fecundating energy of the third as paternal uroboros, we had in mind the overwhelming numinous power of the masculine. But, examined more closely, these three manifestations may also be said to be manifestations of Eros as the dragon-monster. For fecundation, dazzling radiance, and dynamic power are three stages of his efficacy, three forms of his reality.

In this light the "disappearance of Eros" takes on a new and mysterious meaning. On the surface Eros disappears because Psyche has disobeyed his command; on the next deeper level he returns "to the mother," for this is symbolized by the cypress, tree of the Great Mother, in which he sits like a bird, and by his return to captivity, to the palace of Aphrodite. But on the profoundest level we must understand that Eros disappears because Psyche with her lamp could not recognize him for what he "really" is. Subsequently it turns out that Eros reveals his true form to her only gradually, in the course of her own development. His manifestation is dependent on her, he is transformed with Psyche and through her. With each of her labors she apprehends—without knowing it—a new category of his reality.

The labors she performs for him are a rectilinear growth of her consciousness of herself, but also of her awareness of Eros. Precisely because this occurs by degrees, and because she manages not to be destroyed by the overwhelming power of the numinosum that is also Eros, she becomes with each labor more secure and more adequate to the divine power and figure of Eros.

It is with the help of the eagle, the unconscious masculine spirit, that Psyche performs the labor of individuation into which Aphrodite had ironically tricked her. This is the surprising thing about Psyche's development: that it is a development *toward* consciousness that is accompanied throughout *by* consciousness. Yet with her the unconscious forces play a more conspicuous part than in the development of masculine consciousness; the independent activity of Psyche as an ego is less powerful than in the corresponding careers of masculine heroes, as for example those of Heracles or Perseus. But the independent activity of her unconscious wholeness, to which she submits, is all the more compelling.

It is characteristic of the "labors of Psyche" that the component of relatedness, that is, the Eros-component, is increasingly accompanied by a masculine spiritual element, which is at first unconscious but gradually develops into a conscious attitude.

Since we must interpret the action "in terms of the subject," we must understand the helpful animals as powers inside Psyche. But Psyche herself is active, even though her acts are performed by powers within her. Although, as in the creative process, not the ego but inner powers provide the dynamic, there is a certain justification for imputing the act to the individual in whom these powers are at work.

Psyche's process of individuation is a formation of hitherto unformed uroboric powers. At first she lives under the spell of the Eros-dragon, in total unconsciousness, in Bachofen's swamp stage; here the uroboric cycle operates in darkness, broken by no consciousness, disturbed and confused by no illumination. It is "life" as such, a life of drives in the dark, sensual paradise of the dragon, a circle that begins and ends in the darkness of the unconscious. Psyche's act shatters the circle forever. There is an irruption of light and consciousness; the individual relation and love take the place of anonymous lust and the dark embrace of the mere drive.

If we recognize Psyche's development as an archetypal process, the Psyche-Eros constellation becomes the archetype of the relation between man and woman. The phase of their engulfment in the dark paradise of the unconscious corresponds to the initial uroboric situation of psychic existence. It is the phase of psychic identity, in which all things are bound together, fused and inextricably intermingled,[31] as in the state of *participation mystique*. Psychic life is in a phase of dark, that is to say, unconscious mixture, of unconscious stimulation, embrace, and fecundation. And the symbolism of a Psyche united with Eros in the darkness is eminently suited to this universal interrelation of contents in the collective unconscious.

Psyche's act, as we have seen, brings with it a new psychic situation. Love and hate, light and darkness, conscious and unconscious enter into conflict with one another. This is the phase of the separation of the original parents, in which the principle of opposition comes into being. The light of consciousness with its power of analysis and separation breaks into the preceding situation and transforms unconscious identity into a polar relation of opposites. But this opposition was constellated in Psyche's unconscious even before her act; in fact, it has led to her act.

The embrace of Eros and Psyche in the darkness represents the elementary but unconscious attraction of opposites, which impersonally bestows life but is not yet human. But the coming of light makes Eros "visible," it manifests the phenomenon of psychic love, hence of all human love, as the human and higher form of the archetype of relatedness. It is only the completion of Psyche's development, effected in the course of her search for the invisible Eros, that brings with it the highest manifesta-

[31] Cf. my *Origins*, pp. 5 ff.

tion of the archetype of relatedness: a divine Eros joined with a divine Psyche.

Psyche's individual love for Eros as love in the light is not only an essential element, it is *the* essential element in feminine individuation. Feminine individuation and the spiritual development of the feminine—and herein lies the basic significance of this myth—are always effected through love. Through Eros, through her love of him, Psyche develops not only toward him, but toward herself.

The new factor which emerges with the independence of Psyche's love, and which Aphrodite had regarded as impossible, is that a feminine being should have a "stout heart and prudence beyond the prudence of woman." Aphrodite gives no woman credit for these masculine attributes. What is said of Psyche's light-bringing deed is true of Psyche herself. With Psyche, "courage displaced the weakness of her sex." But the unique feature of Psyche's development is that she achieves her mission not directly but indirectly, that she performs her labors with the help of the masculine, but not as a masculine being. For even though she is compelled to build up the masculine side of her nature, she remains true to her womanhood. This is perhaps most clearly shown in the last labor imposed on her by Aphrodite.

In fairy tales and myths the tasks are usually three in number, but in Psyche's case there is characteristically an additional fourth labor. Four is the symbol of wholeness. The first three problems, as we have seen, are solved by "helpers," that is, by inner powers of Psyche's unconscious. But in this last task Psyche herself must do what is asked of her. Hitherto her helpers belonged to the plant and animal world; this time she is sustained by the tower, as symbol of human culture. In her first three tasks Psyche, as we have attempted to show, wrestled with the masculine principle. In her last and fourth task she enters into a direct struggle with the central feminine principle, with Aphrodite-Persephone.

What is here expected of Psyche is neither more nor less than a journey to the underworld. While in the preceding labor Psyche had to take a precious substance from the highest heights, the topmost crag, here the object of her quest is in the lowest depths, in the hands of Persephone herself.

Hitherto we have had to interpret the task in order to understand the helper; here we must take the opposite course. The tower is a symbol on many levels. As mandala-precinct it is feminine: fortress and city and mountain, whose cultural equivalent is the graduated tower and temple tower, the pyramid; it is no accident that the summit of the wall is the crown of the great feminine godhead. But the tower is also phallic as earth phallus: tree, stone, and wall. Aside from this bisexual significance, the tower is an edifice, something erected by human hands, a product of man's collective, spiritual labor; thus it is a symbol of human culture and of the human consciousness and is therefore designated as a "far-seeing tower."

This tower shows Psyche how she as an individual, as woman and human being, can defeat the deadly alliance of the goddesses who, as Aphrodite, Hera, and Demeter, govern the divine-upper sphere and, as Persephone, the divine-lower sphere. In this "extreme journey" Psyche is for the first time herself. No animal can help her, for on this journey nothing and no one can substitute for her.

All alone Psyche undertakes this heroic path of rebirth for the sake of her love, for the sake of Eros, armed with the tower's instructions and the desperate yearning of her heart to find her loved one again in defiance of all obstacles. It had been the eagle's task to carry something human to celestial heights; Psyche must carry something hidden beneath the earth up into the world.

The details of the journey to Persephone need not concern us; the payment of the coin to Charon and the throwing of the sops to Cerberus are traditional motifs, not specific to the story of Psyche. The same is true of the conventional behavior of Persephone. The rule against taking food in the underworld is an archetypal feature of the journey to Hades (we find a parallel in America, for example), without specific bearing on Psyche's journey. But it strikes us as a different matter that Psyche should be forbidden to help the donkey driver, the corpse, and the weaving women.

Here again we may possibly have traditional motifs, but they take on a special significance for Psyche. As the tower teaches Psyche, "pity is not lawful." If, as we shall proceed to show, all Psyche's acts present a rite of initiation, this prohibition implies the insistence on "ego stability" characteristic of every initiation. Among men this stability is manifested as endurance of pain, hunger, thirst, and so forth; but in the feminine sphere it characteristically takes the form of resistance to pity. This firmness of the strong-willed ego, concentrated on its goal, is expressed in countless other myths and fairy tales, with their injunctions not to turn around, not to answer, and the like. While ego stability is a very masculine virtue, it is more; for it is the presupposition of consciousness and of all conscious activity.

The feminine is threatened in its ego stability by the danger of distraction through "relatedness," through Eros. This is the difficult task that confronts every feminine psyche on its way to individuation: it must suspend the claim of what is close at hand for the sake of a distant abstract goal. Thus the tower is perfectly right in saying that these dangers are "snares" set by Aphrodite. The Great Mother, as we recall, also has her life-giving and life-preserving aspect, but in the conflict between Aphrodite and Psyche she reveals only the negative side. This means that here she represents only nature and the species in opposition to the requirements of the individual,[32] and from this standpoint the merciful attitude of the Good Mother can be forbidden to the individual.

The universal component of relatedness is so essential a part of the collective structure of the feminine psyche that Briffault regards it as the foundation of all human community and culture, which he derives from the feminine group with its bond between mothers and children.[33] But this bond is not individual but collective; it pertains to the Great Mother in her aspect as preserver of life, as goddess of fertility, who is not concerned with the individual and individuation, but with the group, which she bids to "be fruitful and multiply."

[32] My *Origins*, pp. 284, 298.
[33] Briffault, *The Mothers*, I, pp. 151 ff.

For this reason the prohibition of pity signifies Psyche's struggle against the feminine nature. Originally "helping" always means a *participation mystique*, which presupposes or creates an identity and is therefore not without danger. It may, for example, lead to a possession by the one who is helped. In the *Thousand and One Nights*, the hero relieves the witch of her burden, and by way of "thanks" she leaps up on his back and cannot be shaken off. And there are countless other examples.

Primitive peoples, as Lévy-Bruhl reports,[34] are not "thankful" to their rescuers or helpers—to doctors, for example—but keep making more and more demands on them. In a sense the rescuer continues to be responsible for the life he has saved, as though it were his own. Help, like eating in common, accepting presents, or being invited to the house of another, establishes a communion. That is why Psyche must refuse Persephone's invitation, for by accepting it she would have fallen into her power. And now let us pass over the remaining details[35] and turn to the central problem of Psyche's last task.

Psyche's mission to seek out Persephone in Hades is a heroic journey which, if successful, will be equivalent to the night sea journey of the sun through the darkness of the underworld. The preceding tasks seemed impossible and might well have been fatal, for example, if

[34] Lévy-Bruhl, *Primitive Mentality*, ch. 11.
[35] The weaving women are a well-known symbol of the Great Mother; the donkey driver is known to us as Aucnus, whose mythical significance has been elucidated by Bachofen; and the corpse who asks Psyche to help him may readily be understood to represent the danger of being possessed by the dead man, by the ancestral spirit.

Psyche had approached the sun rams at noon. Death lurks in every one of the hero's "hard labors," but it is the hardest labor of all that requires direct battle with death or the underworld.

At the outset of every labor Psyche is overcome by a despair in which suicide seems to be the only solution. Now this strange motif falls into a meaningful context. By a surprising turn, the marriage of death to which she had been destined was not consummated, but replaced instead by the dark paradise of Eros. But consummation of the marriage of death, as the oracle of Apollo has proclaimed, is an archetypally given requirement of her relation to Eros. Up to now she has not been conscious of this fact, it has only been manifested in her recurring tendency to suicide. Her journey to Persephone signifies that she must now consciously look death in the face. Now, at the end of her development, she confronts this death situation as one transformed, no longer as an inexperienced girl, but as one who loves, who knows, and who has been tested.

This "extreme journey" becomes possible for Psyche only when, through her labors, she has acquired a consciousness that far transcends the merely instinctive knowledge she possessed to begin with. Thanks to her union with the powers symbolized by the ants, the reed, and the eagle, she is able to adopt the attitude of consciousness that is represented by the "far-seeing tower." Now that Psyche is conscious of her goal; now that she has attained ego stability, she is no longer willing to follow the merely natural demands of her being, and is capable of seeing through the guile of the hostile powers.

She succeeds in returning to the earth because she has assimilated the masculine-spiritual ascending power of the eagle that enables her to rise upward from the darkness and see things "from above." And the symbol of the upreared tower signifies that this is no longer a mere instinctive power, but a "having," a possession.

Psyche is sent by Aphrodite to Persephone, from the goddess of the upper world to the goddess of the lower world; but both are only aspects of the one Great Mother, who is hostile to Psyche. Seldom has the archetypal identification of Aphrodite and Persephone, repeatedly shown in their cults, been made so clear as in this situation.

The splitting up of the primordial archetype into separate goddesses leads to individual cults. The fusion of all the feminine deities into one, as in Apuleius' hymn to Isis, which scholars have mistakenly regarded as the product of a late "syncretistic" conception, is only a late reflection of an authentic primordial context. This is an archetypal fact restricted to no one culture or cultural sphere. The Tibetan Book of the Dead[36] teaches that the favorable and unfavorable gods are only two aspects of the One, and this is the truth. It can be demonstrated for Babylonia and India as well as for Egypt and Greece.

"The nocturnal implications of Aphrodite are profound, although those involving the night of death rather than the night of love are passed over in silence by the classical tradition. Still, we know that in Delphi an Aphrodite 'of the tombs,' an 'Epitymbidia,' was also worshiped. In Greek Lower Italy wonderful monuments

[36] Ed. Evans-Wentz (q.v., List of Works Cited).

of art show us directly how Persephone, the goddess of the underworld, can assume an Aphrodite aspect, and that a profound religious experience was reflected by the Pythagorean belief in two Aphrodites: the one celestial, the other subterranean. Aphrodite also had her Persephone aspect, and where this was known, in the South Italian Greek city of Tarentum, she was called: Queen."[37]

Although the fourth task can be interpreted only against the background of the Eleusinian mysteries and of the Demeter-Kore relationship, which we have examined in another context,[38] we must here give at least some indication of the area in which this episode was enacted.

The content of Psyche's act was that she burst through the matriarchal sphere and in her knowing love of Eros attained the psychic sphere, "the experience of the feminine in encounter," which is the presupposition of feminine individuation. We have recognized Psyche's hostile shadow sisters as matriarchal powers. But with Aphrodite's intervention the conflict was transferred from the personal to the transpersonal plane.

Kore-Persephone and Aphrodite-Demeter are the two great poles and rulers of the central mysteries of the feminine, the Eleusinian mysteries, concerning whose connection with the tale of Psyche we shall have more to say. In her last labor, Psyche finds herself placed between these two poles.

The first three tasks have made it plain that Psyche's

[37] Kerényi, *Töchter*, p. 170.
[38] My *The Great Mother*, pp. 305 ff.

downfall was to be encompassed by the primordial attitude of the matriarchate. Behind the "impossibility" of performing these tasks stood the characteristic matriarchal conception of a negative masculine principle which, Aphrodite had hoped, would prove too much for Psyche. As the labors unfolded, this negative principle was manifested as masculine promiscuity, the deadly masculine, and the uncontainable masculine. Aphrodite's attempt to destroy Psyche in this way reaches its climax in the fourth task.

First we must penetrate the meaning of the box of ointment that Psyche is to bring from Persephone. The task is imposed by Aphrodite, Psyche's mortal enemy; the beauty ointment for which Psyche is sent comes from Persephone; and when Psyche opens the box, she is overcome by a deathlike sleep. Our interpretation is based on these three facts.

The beauty ointment, it seems to us, represents Persephone's eternal youth, the eternal youth of death. It is the beauty of Kore, the beauty of the "deathlike sleep." It is known to us from the tales of Sleeping Beauty and Snow White, where it is also induced by the Bad Mother, the stepmother, or the old witch. It is the beauty of the glass coffin, to which Psyche is expected to regress, the barren frigid beauty of mere maidenhood, without love for a man, as exacted by the matriarchate. This beauty of existence in the unconscious gives the feminine a natural maidenly perfection. But preserved forever, it becomes a beauty of death, a beauty of Persephone, who is inhuman since her existence is one of divine perfection, without fate, suffering, or knowledge. It is Aphrodite's secret aim to make Psyche "die," to make her regress to the Kore-Persephone stage, which was hers before her encounter with Eros.

Here it is the seduction of narcissism that threatens to overpower Psyche. Aphrodite wishes Psyche to regress from the woman who loved Eros, who was "carried away" by her love for him, and to become once more the maiden immured in narcissistic love of herself as in a glass coffin, who sees only herself, and whose womanhood slumbers.[39] To put Persephone's beauty ointment in Psyche's hands is a trick quite worthy of Aphrodite, with her thorough knowledge of womankind. What woman could resist this temptation, and how could a Psyche in particular be expected to resist it?

Psyche "fails," if we may characterize the events beginning with the opening of the box as "Psyche's failure." Heedless of the tower's warning, as formerly of Eros' warning, she opens the box and falls into a death-like sleep. Everything that she had gained up to this point by her arduous acts and sufferings seems lost. Falling into the sleep of death, she returns to Persephone in the manner of Eurydice after Orpheus had turned around. Overpowered by the death aspect of Aphrodite herself, she becomes Kore-Persephone, carried back to the underworld not by Hades, the masculine bridegroom of death, but by the victorious Great Mother as mother of death.

But just as Demeter's intrigue against Hades was not fully successful, because Kore had already entered into

[39] A mythological example for such a regression is the death of Eurydice in the poem of Rilke quoted above (p. 68).

a bond with Hades and eaten of the fertility symbol of the pomegranate, so likewise Aphrodite's attempt to make Psyche regress into the matriarchate is vain. For Psyche is pregnant, and her impregnation by Eros, as will be made clear later on, is the symbol of her profound individual bond with him. Psyche is not concerned with the fertility of nature—which is the only thing that interests Aphrodite—but with the fertility of individual encounter. It is apparent that Psyche's independence begins in the period of her pregnancy. While in the matriarchal sphere pregnancy leads to a reunion of mother and daughter,[40] here Psyche's awakening to the independence that begins with her pregnancy drives her toward her individual relation to Eros, toward love and consciousness.

The happy ending that follows, Eros coming to awaken Psyche, is not a typical "deus ex machina" episode, as it may seem at first sight, but is full of deep meaning and is—if correctly understood—the most ingenious turn in this very ingenious mythical tale.

What has been the cause of Psyche's "failure," why does she "fail" just now, at the end, after she has endured so much and proved herself in so many situations? Is it only an irresistible, deplorable feminine curiosity mingled with vanity that prevents her from fulfilling her mission as messenger in the service of the goddess's cosmetic needs, that impels her to open the box on

[40] Kerényi's observations on the Eleusinian mysteries ("The Psychological Aspects of the Kore") must be completed by a psychological interpretation which shows these feminine mysteries to be the central mysteries of the matriarchal *Weltanschauung*. And see my *The Great Mother*, pp. 305 ff.

which her whole fate depends? Why does Psyche fail, oriented as she is by the far-sighted tower, endowed with a developed consciousness and a stabilized ego that have proved equal to the journey of death into the underworld?

Psyche fails, she must fail, because she is a feminine psyche. But though she does not know it, it is precisely this failure that brings her victory.

One can conceive of no more entrancing form of feminine dragon fight. Elsewhere we have shown that the feminine manner of defeating the dragon is to accept it, and here this insight assumes the surprising but none the less effective form of Psyche's failure. She has traveled the hero's way (we have followed it in all its stages), she has developed a consciousness so strong and radical that through it she has lost her beloved. But now, one step before the end, she disregards the warning of the masculine tower-consciousness and flings herself into the deadly peril that is called Aphrodite-Persephone. And all this for nothing, or next to nothing, all this just to make herself pleasing to Eros.

When Psyche decides to open the box and use the beauty ointment of the goddesses for herself, she must be perfectly well aware of the danger. The tower had warned her urgently enough. Nevertheless she decides not to give what she had acquired with such great pains to the Great Mother, but to steal it.

The story began with the motif of beauty, which now reappears on a new plane. When Psyche was called the new Aphrodite because of her beauty, when she aroused the admiration of men and the jealousy of the goddess, she looked on this gift as a misfortune. But now, just to enhance her beauty, she is willing to take the greatest misfortune on herself. This change in Psyche has occurred for the sake of Eros; it conveys, profoundly though unemphatically, an insight that is not without its tragic aspect.

Psyche is a mortal in a conflict with goddesses; that is bad enough, but since her beloved is also a god, how can she face up to him? She stems from the earthly sphere and aspires to become the equal of her divine lover. In feminine, all too feminine wise, yet not wholly without awareness of her partner's psychology, she seems to say to herself: My acts, my sufferings may move him, may force admiration from him, but soul alone may not be enough. Yet one thing is certain: no Eros will be able to resist a Psyche anointed with divine beauty. So she steals the ointment which confers the beauty that connects Persephone with Aphrodite. And now, when the terrible happens, and the deathlike sleep (which we have interpreted as regression) descends on her—it is no accident that Kore was ravished in the valley that bears the name of the opium poppy[41]—the negative regression which we have seen to be the substance of Psyche's danger seems to set in.

Why does Eros come to save her at just this point, and why are we not willing to agree that this is an appended happy ending? Why do we contend that this is a meaningful and essential part of the whole?

In the beginning Psyche sacrificed her Eros-paradise for the sake of her spiritual development; but now she

[41] See my *The Great Mother*, p. 286.

is just as ready to sacrifice her spiritual development for the immortal beauty of Persephone-Aphrodite, which will make her pleasing to Eros. In so doing, she seems indeed to regress, but it is not a regression to something old, to the matriarchal position, for example. By preferring beauty to knowledge, she reunites herself, rather, with the feminine in her nature. And because she does this lovingly and for Eros, her "old" femininity enters into a new phase. It no longer consists in the self-contained beauty of a young girl who sees nothing beside herself, nor is it the seductive beauty of Aphrodite, who has only the "natural purpose" in mind. It is the beauty of a woman in love, who wishes to be beautiful for the beloved, for Eros, and for no one else.

We have elsewhere shown that centroversion as a tendency toward wholeness is reflected at the primitive level in a general body feeling,[42] and that the body then may be said to represent the totality, the self. The relation to this body-totality is manifested in what has erroneously and negatively been termed "narcissism," an increased emphasis on one's own beauty and wholeness. This phase, which in the masculine development is superseded and replaced by another constellation, is permanently maintained in the woman, whose original relation to the self remains more strongly in force.

In taking so paradoxical a decision at this point, Psyche renews her bond with her feminine center, her self. She professes her love and holds fast to her individual encounter with Eros, but at the same time, in opposition to all—masculine—reason, she discloses her

[42] My *Origins*, p. 307.

primordial femininity. The masculine accent required by her labors is replaced by a feminine accent, and it seems to us that it is just this which, without her knowledge or will, brings her the forgiveness of Aphrodite-Persephone. This, we believe, is the innermost reason why Aphrodite suddenly abandons her opposition and accepts Zeus' deification of Psyche, for Aphrodite, as we know, has often enough resisted the will of Zeus. A Psyche who fails, who for the sake of love renounces all principles, throws all warnings to the winds, and forsakes all reason, such a Psyche must ultimately find favor with Aphrodite, who assuredly recognizes a good part of herself in the new Aphrodite.

This paradoxically feminine failure of Psyche also leads Eros himself to intervene, makes the boy into a man, and transforms the burned fugitive into a savior. By her failure—and this is the profound symmetry of our myth—Psyche has repaired precisely what was undone by the act that drove Eros away. On that occasion, impelled by something that appeared to her as hatred, at the risk of losing Eros she "made light"; now, impelled by a motive that appears to her as love, she is prepared to "make darkness" in order to gain Eros. And it is this situation, in which Psyche, a new Kore-Persephone, sleeps once more in the glass coffin, that gives Eros the possibility of encountering her again on a new plane, as savior and hero. In sacrificing the masculine side, which, necessary as it was, had led to separation, she enters into a situation in which, by her very helplessness and need of salvation, she saves the captive Eros.

Unquestionably Psyche is aware of the danger she is

incurring by opening the box. But here again, and now on a higher plane, she enacts the marriage of death with Eros. She dies for him, she is prepared to give herself and everything she has acquired for him, for—and this is the profound paradox of the situation—with the opening of the box she becomes divinely beautiful in death. The natural naïve beauty and perfection of the maiden who dies in the marriage of death with the male become the knowing, psychic-spiritual beauty of a Psyche who dies for Eros and voluntarily sacrifices her whole being for him.

With this the divine principle undergoes something totally unique and new. Through Psyche's sacrifice and death the divine lover is changed from a wounded boy to a man and savior, because in Psyche he finds something that exists only in the earthly human middle zone between heaven and underworld: the feminine mystery of rebirth through love. In no goddess can Eros experience and know the miracle that befalls him through the human Psyche, the phenomenon of a love which is conscious, which, stronger than death, anointed with divine beauty, is willing to die, to receive the beloved as bridegroom of death.

Now we are also in a position to understand the alliance between Zeus and Eros, resulting in Psyche's reception into heaven. The supreme masculine authority bows to the human and feminine, which by its superiority in love has proved itself equal to the divine.

Thus Psyche's failure is not a regressive, passive sinking, but a dialectical reversal of her extreme activity into devotion. Through the perfection of her femininity and love she calls forth the perfect manhood of Eros. In abandoning herself out of love, she unwittingly achieves redemption through love.

With her redemption by Eros, Psyche has completed her four labors and thus accomplished the initiate's journey through the four elements. But it is characteristic that the feminine Psyche must not simply travel "through" the elements, like the male initiate of the mysteries of Isis; she must make them her own through her acts and sufferings and assimilate them as the helpful forces of her nature: the ants that belong to the earth, the reed that belongs to the water, Zeus' eagle of the air, and finally the fiery, celestial figure of the redeeming Eros himself.

There still remains one point which throws a bright light on Psyche's failure and shows how consequently meaningful it is for the myth as a whole. Once again we can only admire the inner architecture of the myth, which is discernible to the attentive eye despite the idyllic fancies with which it is overgrown.

It is no accident that the scene of Psyche's failure, the place where she opens the box that carries all the associations of Pandora's box of doom, should be the earth. It is only after she has succeeded in returning from the realm of Persephone that Psyche resolves to open the box, but by then she is on her own earthly, human ground, halfway between Aphrodite's heaven and Persephone's underworld.

If she had opened the box in the underworld, the sphere of Persephone's power, there is no doubt that an irremediable catastrophe would have occurred. But the situation is fundamentally changed now that she has returned from the underworld "to the heavenly choir of the stars," now that the treasure has been removed from the underworld. Psyche has taken what she received from Persephone into her own possession; it belongs to her lawfully. Instead of giving up what she has acquired to Aphrodite, she makes it her own; like a feminine Prometheus she, the human Psyche, takes Persephone's treasure for herself. As a human being and an individual, she takes what "properly" belongs to the archetypes, the goddesses, so enacting the deed of the hero, who always incorporates into his own personality the treasure originally guarded and possessed by the dragon of the unconscious. But if Psyche's whole career is interpreted as a process of feminine initiation, the question arises: how are we to understand the role of Aphrodite?

The Aphrodite of our story is not the Great Goddess of classical Greece. She is more and less. More, because behind her we discern the grandiose demonic image of the archaic Terrible Mother; less, because she discloses personalistic traits more reminiscent of a human home life molded by terrible mothers than of a divine reality.

We know that the Great Mother may appear as a figure of the feminine self.[43] To what extent, we must ask then, does Aphrodite play the part of the self in our tale, or rather, to what extent does the self use the archetype of the Great Mother for its purposes?[44]

[43] Cf. my *The Great Mother*, p. 336.
[44] We find the same problem in the myth of Demeter and Kore, where Gaea beyond any doubt favors the abduction of

In the life of the masculine hero, which we have analyzed elsewhere,[45] we encounter the relation of the self to the parent archetype in a similar situation. The hero is frequently opposed by the negative parent archetype, often personalized as the Bad Father or Bad Mother, but also in the archetypal form of a divine persecutor. The best known example of this constellation is, as we have said, the relation between Hera and Heracles. But as Hera spurs on the hero to his heroism, so here too Aphrodite drives Psyche to her act. Seen from this aspect, the "bad, persecuting" archetype shifts into the archetype that sets development in motion and so promotes individuation. For Psyche, then, there is not only a negative unity of Aphrodite-Persephone, but also the superior though still nameless unity of a Great Goddess as guiding Sophia-Self, one aspect of whom is represented by Aphrodite as Terrible Mother, who keeps "sending her on her way."

Here the contrast between the masculine and feminine view of the archetypal feminine becomes clear, and it is a contrast that belongs to the psychic background of Apuleius' book. Aphrodite-Fortuna was the *heimarmene* of that period; she was "bad fortune" and Terrible Mother, in opposition to Isis, who as Good Mother and Sophia was the goddess of the "good fortune" transformed by the mystery. It is in the light of this opposition that the feminine appears to a masculine psychology, and so also to Apuleius in his final chapter on the

---

Kore, so that an antagonism between Gaea and Demeter is evident.

[45] My *Origins*, pp. 131 ff.

initiation into the rite of Isis. But this is not so for Psyche herself, this "incarnation" of the feminine and its psychology.

The conception of the archetypal feminine as a unity is one of woman's fundamental experiences. The ancient pantheon with its antithetical goddesses still represented this conception, but in the patriarchal world it was dissolved. In the patriarchate the split into the Good and the Bad Mother caused the negative side of the feminine to be thrust back very largely into the unconscious. And moreover, precisely because this splitting-off of a "bad" from a "good" feminine archetype was only partially successful, the goddess was entirely banished from heaven, as in the patriarchal monotheistic religions. The deification of the human Psyche in our myth represents a kind of countermovement to this degradation of the goddesses.

But Psyche's experience of the unity of the archetypal feminine is not the primitive experience of opposites still joined in numinously uroboric unity; it is the experience of totality, which woman in her individuation incurs as a product of her own process of becoming whole.

Here it should be stressed that the myth of Psyche *is* archetypal and in this sense historically paradigmatic; it announces a development that had not yet taken place in the individual man of antiquity. Psyche herself does not come consciously to her experience of the archetypal feminine as a unity, but this experience is the effective reality behind her development.

We have seen that in Aphrodite the figure of the Bad Mother is merged with that of the feminine self as Sophia, driving toward individuation. But the connection between Great Mother, the psychology of the matriarchate, the role of the sisters, the feminine self, must be further clarified and interpreted, although we cannot discuss the entire problem of the primordial feminine relation, the relation between mother and daughters.[45a]

In its development the feminine personality must pass through a number of phases, each of which is characterized by definite archetypal phenomena. The development runs from the original situation, with its far-reaching identity of mother-daughter-self-ego, by way of the matriarchate, in which, despite the greater freedom and independence of the ego, the archetype of the Great Mother is still dominant, and by way of the paternal uroboros, to the patriarchate, in which the dominance of the Great Mother archetype gives way to that of the Great Father. This situation of the patriarchate—known to us particularly from its Western development—is characterized by a recession of feminine psychology and its dominants; now feminine existence is almost entirely determined by the masculine world of consciousness and its values.

The collective phase of the patriarchate with its subordination of the feminine gives way to the phase of "encounter," in which the masculine and the feminine confront each other individually. Then, in the phase of individuation, woman frees herself from the decisive in-

[45a] See my *The Great Mother*, pp. 305 f.

fluence of encounter with the masculine and is guided by the experience of her self as a feminine self.[46]

The self stands for wholeness. Not only does it tend in centroversion[47] toward the formation of the ego and consciousness, but it goes further toward individuation, in which the self is experienced as the center of wholeness. When the unconscious forces of a phase that is being transcended resist the ego and the development of individuation, we always have a conflict between the unconscious as Great Mother, holding fast to that which is born from her, and the self which tends toward the development of wholeness.

Now it is an essential difficulty of feminine psychology that the feminine must develop toward and beyond the masculine, which represents consciousness over against the unconscious. Herein it comes into conflict with the Great Mother, the feminine archetype of the unconscious, and with the primordial feminine relation as exemplified in the myth of Demeter and Kore. But this development in conflict with the Great Mother must not lead to a violation of the feminine nature by the masculine and its peculiar psychology; nor must it cause woman to lose contact with the unconscious and the feminine self. The difficulty of distinguishing between the progressive character of the self and the regressive

[46] This schematic representation of the development does not, of course, correspond to the reality, in which there is no rectilinear development. Moreover, a new phase does not simply replace the preceding phase, but forms a new level in the psychic structure, which had hitherto been determined by the other phases and their laws.

[47] My *Origins*, pp. 261 ff.

character of the Great Mother is one of the central problems not only of feminine psychology.[48]

In Psyche's development the psychology of the matriarchate is represented by the sisters, who symbolize the sister bond of the feminine group and at the same time its hostility toward the personal man. Matriarchal hostility toward encounter with the man, that is, toward love, must indeed be overcome, and the patriarchate represents a necessary transition stage even for feminine development, but "imprisonment in the patriarchate," "harem psychology," is a regression over against the matriarchal independence of womanhood. For this reason an essential and positive element is contained in the opposition of the matriarchal powers to the imprisonment of the feminine in the patriarchate as well as its servitude to the Eros-dragon, the paternal uroboros.

In this sense "regression" to the matriarchal powers often has a progressive meaning, as may be ascertained in the psychology of modern woman. Even if the powers represent a part of the feminine shadow, their assimilation, as in the case of Psyche's act, may lead to a new integration and a broadening of the personality.

This, however, occurs only when the powers are accepted in favor of a still unknown and broadened personality, a movement toward psychic wholeness, and not when the psyche surrenders to a destructive, personally regressive shadow aspect such as the sisters represent in the tale of Psyche. The negativity of the sisters is already manifested in the negative designs of their consciousness with regard to Psyche; it becomes perfectly

[48] My "Die mythische Welt und der Einzelne."

clear when we consider their subsequent development—if their doom may be called a development. Significant psychological and mythological elements are concealed in this episode, which is represented as the vengeance of Eros and Psyche on the sisters. At the risk of being suspected of an over-interpretation, we shall point out these connections, although their full significance can be disclosed only by an exposition of feminine development in all its phases.

The death of the sisters through Eros is a typical example of the destruction of the feminine through the paternal uroboros. Unconsciously the sisters are as much possessed by Psyche's lover as she herself, if not more so. They take him for a god almost at once and rightly associate with him the sensual paradise that Psyche really experiences with Eros. The fascination by this divine lover is highly "personalized" in the tale, for palace, gold, jewels, and so forth appear here as "earthly" attractions, but behind them the power of the suprapersonal fascination by Eros is still discernible. We must not forget the situation of these sisters, captives to patriarchal marriage, pining away in the role of daughterly or motherly sick-nurses. Despite their comic aspect, their envy and malignant hate-jealousy of Psyche, as well as their headlong readiness to abandon everything and fling themselves into the arms of Eros, they are not without a secret tragic quality. Their end, characteristically, is wholly mythical. In their feverish hallucination they leap down from a cliff, the classical cliff of the bride of death, where Psyche had stood—and are dashed to pieces. In the uncanny justice of the myth, the blinded sisters with their madness bear witness to the truth of all the negative statements they had made to Psyche regarding her invisible lover, and in a darkly tragic way replace Psyche in the fulfillment of her death. For them Eros is really the devouring masculine monster, the grim beast of the Pythian oracle. Beyond their man-murdering consciousness, they are seized by Eros in the manner of Dionysian maenads; it is in amorous frenzy that they fling themselves off the cliff. They are true parallels to the women who are unconsciously seized by Dionysus in attempting to resist him, and who die in maenadic madness.

But in the course of her development Psyche has freed herself both from the matriarchal powers which had given her her revolutionary impetus and from captivity in the sensual paradise that Eros as paternal uroboros had offered her. The help of the feminine—of Demeter-Hera—was denied Psyche and she has been compelled to travel the masculine road, on which she had started with dagger and lamp, to the bittersweet end. With the invisible assistance of Pan she has performed the matriarchal tasks set her by Aphrodite; and this means that in her encounter with Eros she has gone forward to strata of her unconscious in which masculine powers and figures are dominant.

The masculine powers in the feminine unconscious extend far beyond the so-called "animus" figures.[49] They include uroboric forms that exceed the "purely mascu-

[49] Jung, "The Relations between the Ego and the Unconscious," pp. 186 ff.

line,"[50] as well as extrahuman configurations. In the feminine unconscious animals such as the serpent, but also the bull, ram, horse, and so forth, symbolize the still-primitive fructifying power of the masculine spirit, and the birds, from the fructifying spirit-doves to Zeus' eagle, are likewise symbols of such spiritual powers, as the rites and myths of all peoples show. The fructifying masculine in the vegetable world, for example, as eaten fruit, is archetypally just as effective as the inorganic power of the stones or the wind, which like every fructifying principle always bears a spiritual element within it. This anonymous masculine spiritual principle, with its productive and destructive side, this principle that we designate as the paternal uroboros, represents a psychic power which operates at the fringe of the animus world of the feminine, and beyond it.

With her first three acts Psyche set in motion the knowledge-bringing masculine-positive forces of her nature. But, in addition, she converted the unconscious forces that had helped her into conscious activity and so liberated her own masculine aspect. Her way, consciously traveled by the ego in opposition to the Great Mother, is the typical career of the masculine hero, at the end of which Psyche would have been transformed into a Nike. A very questionable triumph, as feminine developments in this direction have sufficiently shown. For to achieve such a victorious masculine development at the price of her erotic attraction—that is, her attraction for Eros— would have been a catastrophe for a feminine Psyche, whose actions were undertaken for love, that is, under

[50] My "Über den Mond."

the sign of Eros. This outcome is prevented by what we have interpreted as "Psyche's failure."

After becoming conscious of her masculine components and realizing them, and having become whole through development of her masculine aspect, Psyche was in a position to confront the totality of the Great Mother in her twofold aspect as Aphrodite-Persephone. The end of this confrontation was the paradoxical victory-defeat of Psyche's failure, with which she regained not only an Eros transformed into a man, but also her contact with her own central feminine self.

At this point Psyche is received into Olympus, guided upward by Hermes, deified, and united forever with Eros. Here Hermes once more fulfills his true and proper function as *psychopompos*, guide of souls. As he served Aphrodite in the beginning, he was nothing more than the "messenger of the gods," the secondary and easily caricatured figure of the Roman pantheon. But now that Psyche attains the immortality she has earned, Hermes too is redeemed, regaining his primal mythical form; his true hermetic efficacy as guide of the feminine soul becomes discernible.

When Psyche is received into Olympus as the wife of Eros, an epoch-making development of the feminine and of all humanity is manifested in myth. Seen from the feminine standpoint, this signifies that the soul's individual ability to love is divine, and that transformation by love is a mystery that deifies. This experience of the feminine psyche takes on special importance against the background of the ancient patriarchal world with its

collective feminine existence, subordinated to the rule of
the fertility principle.

The human has conquered its place on Olympus, but
this has been done not by a masculine deified hero, but
by a loving soul. Human womanhood as an individual
has mounted to Olympus, and here, in the perfection
achieved by the mystery of love, woman stands beside the
archetypes of mankind, the gods. And paradoxically
enough, she has gained this divine place precisely by her
mortality. It is the experience of mortality, the passage
through death to rebirth and resurrection to Eros, that
makes Psyche divine in a mystery of transformation that
carries her beyond the inhumanity of the "only godly"
as conceived by the ancients.

In this connection we are enabled to understand a
last problem, that of the child born of Psyche's union
with Eros. This child, whose growth accompanies Psyche's whole development and calvary, is first mentioned
just as Psyche discloses the early stirrings of independence.
After the first visit of the sisters, Eros tells Psyche of her
pregnancy and utters the mysterious words: "Your
womb, a child's as yet, bears a child like to you. If you
keep my secret in silence, he shall be a god; if you divulge it, a mortal."

What can these words mean? Are we taking them too
seriously in supposing that they must be interpreted?
For after all Psyche *does* bear a divine child, and it
would seem at first sight that she scarcely kept the
"secret" silent—assuredly not if Eros' invisibility was
its substance. Since we must exclude this interpreta-

tion, the question rises: what was the secret that Psyche must not profane?

The true and ineffable mystery, the "secret" that must not be "divulged" and profaned, consists in Psyche's inner loyalty to Eros, the loyalty of the human Psyche to her mysterious and "impossible" love, and to the essential transformation that she undergoes through her relationship with her divine partner. For from a "profane" point of view, as seen by Aphrodite and everyone else, this love is an absurdity and a paradox; it is something both forbidden and impossible. The true secret is observed by Psyche even in opposition to Eros himself and over his resistance, for the ineffable secret of her love is expressible only through Psyche's life, through her acts and transformation. Although Psyche blurts out everything that can possibly be blurted out, this innermost kernel of her love retains its efficacy as an unuttered secret within her. Even Eros himself is enabled to discern it only through Psyche's self-sacrifice, for the understanding of what love and its true secret are becomes accessible to him, becomes living experience for him, only through Psyche's love. Hitherto he had experienced love only in the darkness, as a wanton game, as an onslaught of sensual desire in the willing service of Aphrodite; but through Psyche's act he experiences it as a travail of the personality, leading through suffering to transformation and illumination.

Marriage of death, existence in the paradise of the unconscious, fight with the dragon, calvary of labors, journey to the underworld and acquisition of the precious substance, failure as second death (which in myth often takes the form of imprisonment),[51] redemption, *hieros gamos*, resurrection, rebirth as a goddess, and birth of the child—these are not separate archetypal motifs; they represent the whole canon of archetypes, which runs not only through myths and fairy tales, but occurs in the mysteries as well, and has also disclosed countless variants of its basic structure in the religious systems, in Gnosticism for example. This mystery career does not consist only in action; usually its meaning lies in the growth of knowledge, of gnosis. But here (as in the Eleusinian mysteries) it takes a specifically different form. It is not a mystery of gnosis, that is, of the logos, but a mystery of Eros. And accordingly the child who is born, contrary to the expectations of Eros,[52] is a girl.

In her love for Eros, Psyche is not only different from Aphrodite or any other goddess; she is something wholly new. The triumph of Psyche's love and her ascension to Olympus were an event that has profoundly affected Western mankind for two thousand years. For two millenniums the mystery phenomenon of love has occupied the center of psychic development and of culture, art, and religion. The mysticism of the medieval nuns, the courtly love of the troubadours, Dante's love for Beatrice, Faust's Eternal Feminine—all reflect this never-resting mystery-like development of the psyche in woman and man. It has brought both good and evil, but in any event it has been an essential ferment of the

[51] My *Origins*, p. 319.
[52] Weinreich, "Das Märchen von Amor und Psyche," in Friedländer, *Darstellungen aus der Sittengeschichte Roms.* See Apuleius' tale, p. 18, above.

psychic and spiritual life of the West down to the present day.

This love of Psyche for her divine lover is a central motif in the love mysticism of all times, and Psyche's failure, her final self-abandonment, and the god who approaches as a savior at this very moment correspond exactly to the highest phase of mystical ecstasy, in which the soul commends itself to the godhead.

For this reason it is said that "in the language of mortals" Psyche's child "is called Pleasure." But in the language of heaven—and it is a heavenly child whom the deified Psyche bears in heaven—this child is the mystical joy which among all peoples is described as the fruit of the highest mystical union. It is "Joy indeed, but surpassing sensuality."[53]

The "birth of the divine child" and its significance are known to us from mythology, but even more fully from what we have learned of the individuation process.[54] While to a woman the birth of the divine son signifies a renewal and deification of her animus-spirit aspect, the birth of the divine daughter represents a still more central process, relevant to woman's self and wholeness.

It is one of this myth's profoundest insights that makes it end with the birth of a daughter who is Pleasure-Joy-Bliss. This last sentence relating the transcendent birth of the daughter, which actually surpasses the myth itself, suggests a corner of inner feminine experience

[53] Tejobindu Upanishad 8 (in Deussen, *Sechzig Upanishad's*, p. 665).

[54] Cf. Jung's works, *The Secret of the Golden Flower*, "The Psychology of the Child Archetype," *Psychology and Alchemy*, etc.

which defies description and almost defies understanding, although it is manifested time and time again as the determining borderline experience of the psyche and of psychic life.

We have repeatedly stressed that this tale embodies a *myth*, that is to say, a complete, self-contained action "in archetypal space." Precisely because it is an archetypal action, its meaning must be taken in a collective human sense and not personalistically, that is, not as something that takes place in a particular man or a particular woman, but as a universal "exemplary action."

Here it will not be possible to describe the psychological difference between the "Psyche-archetype" and that of the anima in man, or of the feminine self in woman. A few indications may suffice. It is no accident that we speak of the "soul" of man as well as woman;[55] and it is no accident that analytical psychology defines the totality of consciousness and the unconscious as the "psyche." This psyche as the whole of the personality must be characterized in man as well as in woman as feminine, because it experiences that which transcends the psychic as numinous, as "outside" and "totally different." For this reason, the mandala figure, which appears in man and woman as the totality of the psyche, is feminine in its symbolism as circle and round, or uroboric as that which contains the opposites.

Where this psyche undergoes experience, the symbolically masculine structure of the ego and of consciousness seems, both in man and woman, to be so rela-

[55] In contrast to the "soul-image" *in* the man and *in* the woman.

tivized and reduced that the feminine character of psychic life is predominant. Thus the mystical birth of the godhead in the man does not take place as birth of the anima, i.e., of a partial structure of psychic life, but as birth of the totality, i.e., of the psyche.[56]

What in the myth of Psyche is born as a daughter is something that transcends the psychic; it is an emotional reality, a metapsychic situation that is constellated when the human psyche is united with its divine partner. And thus the secular meaning of Psyche's deification is disclosed from a new angle.

The situation of the mortal Psyche was this: she seemed to be at the mercy of a hostile world of archetypal feminine powers; Eros clung without independence to these powers, whose incarnation was Aphrodite; and Zeus, the father archetype, stood aside, inactive. From a psychological point of view, this means that the world of the unconscious, in its inhuman, antihuman constellation, dominated human action, and that man's relation to this world—Eros—was also wholly passive. The psychic aspect of the human was utterly at the mercy of the gods and their whims.

But in the myth Psyche is so active that all actions and transformations start with her; she performs a decisive act while Eros sleeps and completes her labors while Eros lies wounded in his mother's house; she, the earthborn woman, succeeds in integrating the four earthly elements of her nature and so in resisting all the intrigues

[56] This variation on Jung's definition of the anima strikes me as a necessary consequence of Jung's own observations of the individuation process.

of the unconscious and its goddess. So great is Psyche's inner strength, so great is her power of integration, acquired through suffering and love, that she can stand up to the disintegrating power of the archetypes and confront them on an equal footing. Yet all this does not occur in a Promethean-masculine opposition to the divine, but in a divine, erotic seizure of love, which shows her to be even more deeply rooted in the center of the divine Aphrodite.

While formerly, as an ancient representation shows us,[57] Aphrodite literally rode on Psyche, or in other words, the archetype of the Great Mother dominated Psyche, Psyche has now been deified through her capacity for love and is borne aloft by Hermes. Through her ascension to Olympus she demonstrates that a new epoch has begun. That Psyche has become a goddess means that the human is itself divine and equal to the gods; and the eternal union of the goddess Psyche with the god Eros means that the human bond with the divine is not only eternal, but itself of a divine quality.

The psychic turn of the divine, the inward journey of the gods into what we call the human psyche, within which this divine principle now appears, has its archetypal beginning in this apotheosis of Psyche.

Strangely enough, the tale of Psyche thus represents a development which in an extra-Christian area, without revelation and without church, wholly pagan and yet transcending paganism, symbolizes the transformation and deification of the psyche. It was another fifteen hundred years before it again became possible and meaning-

[57] See in Reitzenstein, *Das Märchen von Amor und Psyche.*

ful, under entirely new circumstances, to speak of a deification of the human psyche. It was only after the medieval ban on the feminine-earthly side of psychic life—a ban laid down by a spiritual world one-sidedly oriented toward celestial-masculine values—began to be lifted that the divine in earthly nature and the human soul could be rediscovered.[58] Thus in the modern era a new development of the feminine set in, just as, with the rise of depth psychology, a new form of psychic development and transformation is beginning to be discernible in the West.

All these developments are realizations of what is exemplified on an archetypal plane in the myth of Psyche and her deification. Thus it may not be without meaning that this work on Eros and Psyche should appear at the very moment when the Catholic Church, with the dogma of Mary's physical assumption into heaven, is repeating, renewing, and confirming what was enacted in the person of Psyche on the pagan Olympus.[59]

The archetype of Psyche united with Eros, taken together with the child of Joy, strikes us as one of the highest forms that the symbol of the *coniunctio* has taken in the West. It is the youthful form of Shiva united with his Shakti. The hermaphrodite of alchemy is a later but

[58] See my "Die Bedeutung des Erdarchetyps für die Neuzeit," *EJ 1953*.

[59] To the Christian Trinity corresponds the "trinitarian duality" of Zeus and Eros, who in his highest stage of manifestation as winged Eros possesses the character both of Son and Holy Ghost; and the figure of Psyche is analogous to Mary. The psychological meaning of the difference between the ancient Hellenistic and the modern Christian tetrads cannot concern us here.

lesser form of this image, because, as Jung has pointed out, it actually represents a monstrosity, contrasting sharply with the divine pair, Eros and Psyche.

From the standpoint of the feminine, Psyche eternally united with Eros is the feminine self joined with the masculine godhead. Here the accent lies on Psyche, who experiences the transcendent figure of Eros as the luminous aspect of the redeeming logos in herself, through which she attains to illumination and deification. In conceptual simplification, this means that she experiences Eros as gnosis, through love.

From the masculine standpoint, Psyche united with Eros is again the union of the psyche as the totality of the male personality (as known to us, for example, from the archetype of the mandala) with the transcendent masculine-divine manifestation of the self. But for the masculine the accent is less on Psyche than on the divine Eros. Here the transformation of the masculine logos aspect leads to a principle of divine love, which joins with the psyche to produce illumination and deification. Or, in conceptual simplification, the masculine experiences Eros as love, through gnosis.

The interweaving of these two divine figures and mystical experiences constitutes the archetype of the *coniunctio* of Eros and Psyche. Their gloriole, and at the same time the supreme fruit of their union, whose earthly reflection is pleasure, is their divine child, heavenly bliss.

When we survey the development of Psyche as a whole, it becomes clear—and it is already apparent from the connection between the tale and Apuleius' novel in which it is set—that this mythical tale represents a mystery action. What is this mystery action and what position does it occupy in Apuleius' *Golden Ass?*

From the initiation of Lucius Apuleius into the rite of Isis, with which the novel ends, we learn[60] the essential elements of the mystery. The rite consists in a voluntary death and a redemption from death through grace—the journey to the realm of Persephone and back again. It centers in the vision and cult of the upper and lower gods; and significantly it begins with a journey to Hades and a passage through the four elements. (For the present we shall disregard the final stage, that of the transformation in Helios.)

The correspondences with the myth of Psyche are obvious; we cannot but assume that Apuleius knew exactly what he was doing in including the tale in the *Golden Ass.* Our next question is: what is the relation of the story of Psyche to the initiation rite described in the novel?

Here we cannot dispense with a few additional remarks about matriarchal and patriarchal psychology, for it is the conflict between them that makes the myth of Psyche intelligible. Contrasting with the solemn initiation, which is described with all the pomp and ceremony of the mystery terminology, the tale is a profane interpolation. It is conceived as a sort of folkloristic prologue.

In the *Golden Ass* the story of Eros and Psyche is related by an old woman to a young girl. On her wedding day this girl had been snatched "from her mother's

[60] Dibelius, "Die Isisweihe bei Apuleius und verwandte Initiations-Riten."

{ 146 }

arms" by robbers who wished to extort a ransom from her parents. The motif of rape and marriage of death, as well as that of feminine initiation, is discernible in the veiled form characteristic of Apuleius.

The tale of Psyche, which the old woman tells the young bride by way of consolation, is an initiation into the feminine destiny of development through suffering, for it is only after misfortune and suffering that Psyche is reunited with her beloved. That this old woman comes from Thessaly, the land of witches and of Hecate, that is, the land of Pheraia,[61] the great pre-Hellenic Mother Goddess, broadens the background and gives us a glimpse of the matriarchal mysteries in their mythical depth.

It was Bachofen who first gained an intimation of these contexts. To be sure, he forced the tale into his schema and dealt most arbitrarily with the text, which under the circumstances he was bound to misunderstand. But even so, he recognized the story's trend and mystery character. "The feminine soul, first in the service of Aphrodite, a slave to matter, condemned at every step to new and unexpected sufferings, and finally led down into the deepest morass of sensuality—but then arising to a new and more powerful existence, passing from Aphrodisian to Psychic life. The lower phase bears a tellurian, the higher a uranian character. . . . In Psyche Aphrodite herself attains to the lunar stage, the highest which woman's materiality can attain. Beside her stands Eros as Lunus."[62]

[61] Philippson, *Thessalische Mythologie.*
[62] *Versuch über die Gräbersymbolik,* p. 46.

He failed to perceive the conflict between Psyche and Aphrodite or the independently feminine character of the myth, for the great discoverer and admirer of the matriarchate remained hampered by Platonic, Christian, patriarchal conceptions. He could apprehend the feminine-psychic principle only as a stage subordinated to solar-masculine spirituality.

With his Platonizing interpretation and disregard of the myth's details, Bachofen could recognize only a very general "purification" of the soul in the tale of Psyche. He speaks of the details as "legendary motifs" (as though this meant anything other than archetypal traits) and loses himself in vague generalities. Such an interpretation fails to note what is most essential to this myth and tale, namely the feminine psychology with its crises, decisions, and specifically feminine activity.

Contrary to Bachofen, we believe that a myth of the feminine is discernible in the tale of Psyche. And if this is so, it means that we have here a later and higher stage of feminine initiation than that embodied in the Eleusinian mysteries.

In psychological terms the Eleusinian mysteries, like those of Isis, are matriarchal mysteries that differ essentially from the masculine-patriarchal mystery. The masculine mystery is bound up with the active heroic struggle of the ego and based on the central insight that "I and the father are one."[63] But the primordial feminine mysteries have a different structure. They are mysteries of birth and rebirth and appear predominantly in three different forms: as birth of the logos, son of light;

[63] My *Origins*, pp. 265 f.

as birth of the daughter, the new self; and as birth of the dead in rebirth. Wherever we find this elementary feminine symbolism, we have—psychologically speaking —matriarchal mysteries, regardless of whether those initiated are men or women.

While the masculine mysteries start from the priority of the spirit and look upon the reality of the phenomenal world and of matter as the creation of the spirit, the feminine mysteries start from the priority of the phenomenal, "material" world, from which the spiritual is "born."[64] In this sense the patriarchal mysteries are upper and heavenly, while those of the feminine seem lower and chthonian; in the patriarchal mysteries the accent is on the generative numinosity of the invisible. The two are complementary, and it is only taken together that they yield an approach to the whole truth of the mystery.

Psychologically speaking, it is by no means indifferent whether a man is initiated into matriarchal mysteries or a woman into patriarchal mysteries, or the reverse. The masculine may be initiated into matriarchal mysteries in two essentially different ways, both of which lead to entirely different psychic developments than the "patriarchal mystery" of the father-son relationship.

The one way consists in identification with the born son, that is, a return to the mystery of the mother archetype; the second is identification with the feminine, involving a self-abandonment of the masculine. (Here it need not concern us whether this loss is symbolized in real castration, in the tonsure, in the drinking of a medi-

[64] See my *The Great Mother*, pp. 281 f.

cine that renders impotent, or in the adoption of feminine dress.)

If we now return to Lucius and the mystery of Isis, we understand that his "solification," his transformation into Sun-Light-God, is at the same time a transformation into the son of Isis, into Horus-Osiris or Harpocrates, who is born and reborn by the grace of the Great Mother Goddess.

At all events, it is the feminine which assumes the guidance in the redemption of Lucius by Isis and his initiation into her mysteries. It was the evil goddess of fate who stood behind the metamorphosis of Lucius into an ass and all his sufferings, and now it is a good goddess of fate, as Sophia-Isis, greatest of the goddesses, who takes possession of him and leads him to salvation.[65] And here—almost imperceptibly—a new link is forged between the initiation and the tale of Psyche.

In the tale the course of events is also determined through the activity of the feminine partner, of Psyche. The transformations of Eros, Eros as dragon, Eros as monster and husband, Eros as sleeper, and finally Eros as redeeming god who awakens Psyche to supreme being—these stages are attained not by the efforts of Eros himself, but by Psyche's acts and sufferings. It is always *she* who undertakes, suffers, performs, and com-

[65] Here we cannot go into the question of whether the *Golden Ass* throws any light on the authenticity or inauthenticity of Apuleius' experience of initiation: whether the novel is characteristic only of the psychology of this period, when "everyone" was "always" undergoing initiation; or whether Apuleius' narrative points to a psychologically authentic process of transformation.

pletes, and even the manifestation of the divine, of Eros, is ultimately induced by the loving and knowing activity of the feminine aspect, of the human Psyche.

In Eros as in Lucius, the development at every stage starts not from the activity of the masculine ego, but from the initiative of the feminine. In both cases the process—for good and evil—is carried out by this feminine principle, in opposition to a resisting and passive masculine ego. And such developments, in which "the spontaneity of the psyche" and its living guidance are the crucial determinants in the life of the masculine, are known to us from the psychology of the creative process and of individuation. In all these processes where "Psyche leads" and the masculine follows her,[66] the ego relinquishes its leading role and is guided by the totality. In psychic developments which prove to be centered round the nonego, the self, we have creative processes and processes of initiation in one.

While in the tale of Psyche the myth of feminine individuation leads to the supreme union of the feminine with the divine lover, Apuleius' novel, as though to complement this feminine initiation with a masculine one, ends with the introduction of Lucius into the mystery of Isis, where the Great Mother manifests herself as Sophia and the Eternal Feminine.

Apuleius prays to the Goddess: "Holiest of the Holy, perpetual comfort of mankind, you whose bountiful grace nourishes the whole world; whose heart turns to-

[66] These developments are best known to us where the masculine is led by a partial structure of the psyche, a partial aspect of its directive totality, namely the anima.

wards all those in sorrow and tribulation as a mother's to her children. . . . The gods above adore you, the gods below do homage to you, you set the orb of heaven spinning around the poles, you give light to the sun, you govern the universe, you trample down the powers of Hell. At your voice the stars move, the seasons recur, the spirits of earth rejoice, the elements obey." And he concludes: "I will keep your divine countenance always before my eyes and the secret knowledge of your divinity locked deep in my heart."[67]

In these lines we perceive a magnificent prefiguration of a song composed almost two thousand years later, a song that is full of the voice and image of Psyche:

> *Blicket auf zum Retterblick*
> *Alle reuig Zarten,*
> *Euch zu seligem Geschick*
> *Dankend umzuarten.*
> *Werde jeder bessre Sinn*
> *Dir zum Dienst erbötig;*
> *Jungfrau, Mutter, Königin,*
> *Göttin, bleibe gnädig.*[68]

---

[67] Tr. Robert Graves.

[68] [Goethe, *Faust*, Part II, closing scene. — "Look up to the saving look, all ye tender penitents, and so in thankfulness remold yourselves to a blissful destiny. Thee let every better nature be ready to serve; Maid, Mother, Queen, Goddess, still be thou gracious!" (Tr. Willard R. Trask.)]

POSTSCRIPT

THE STORY of Amor and Psyche transmitted to us in the *Golden Ass* was not the invention of Apuleius. What was narrated in the form of a tale by Apuleius, born in A.D. 124, actually originated in a much earlier day.[1]

Like almost all folk tales, this one contains mythical substance that was excluded from the mythology recognized by the dominant culture. The Egyptian tale of Bata, for example, has preserved the original myth of Isis and Osiris. But the tale of Psyche is unique in far more than this. The most fascinating aspect of it is that, along with its abundance of mythical traits and contexts, it represents a development whose content is precisely the liberation of the individual from the primordial mythical world, the freeing of the psyche.

The scholarship of recent years has disclosed a wealth of actual and possible sources and influences which seem to have converged in the tale of Psyche. But this discussion is only of secondary interest to us. What concerns the psychologist is not so much the origin and history of the parts as the meaningful unity of the whole in relation to its parts.

But just as we can often arrive at the meaning of a dream only by an amplification of its parts, so an understanding of the new synthesis of the traditional material

[1] Fulgentius tells us that Apuleius borrowed the tale from the Athenian storyteller Aristophontes, but this is no more helpful to us than the fact that art works of the classical period show familiarity with the story. Rohde, *Der griechische Roman und seine Vorläufer*, p. 371 n.

throws light on the meaning of the whole. It is neither surprising nor very illuminating that comparative research should have disclosed a large number of folktale motifs in the tale of Psyche,[2] for this only means that the same archetypal motifs occur in different places. And the question of whether we have to do with a migration or with a spontaneous reappearance of these motifs is irrelevant for our purposes.

It has been said that in this tale "the destiny of the human soul purified by diverse trials is represented after the model of the Platonic allegories."[3] There is no doubt a certain banal truth in this statement, but taken as a generalization it is just as false as the confusion between Platonic symbols and allegories.

Like all interpretations that disregard the complexity and originality of the Psyche myth, this one, which makes Apuleius' Platonism responsible for the whole tale, must be rejected. Still, there is no doubt that a tradition transmitted by Plato played an important part in shaping the myth, and of this we shall have more to say below.

Yet it is equally absurd to speak of an "ethical purpose" in the *Golden Ass*, which has not yet become clear in the tale of Psyche.[4] Here, as so often, Bachofen intuitively[5] perceived and interpreted highly important relationships. It is true that we agree with him only in certain points, because we are no longer hampered by the Christian-ethical dogmatism of Bachofen's time, and

[2] Weinreich, "Das Märchen von Amor und Psyche," in Friedländer, *Darstellungen aus der Sittengeschichte Roms*.

[3] Ilmer, *Einleitung zu Apuleius, Der Goldene Esel*, p. iii.

[4] Ibid., p. iv.

[5] *Versuch über die Gräbersymbolik.*

take the insights of depth psychology as our starting point. Be that as it may, Bachofen was the first writer to see that the story of Psyche reflects an important sector of feminine-psychic development. In this connection we must bear in mind the magnificent passage in Bachofen's "Mother Right,"[6] where he equates Eros with Dionysus and derives certain basic situations of feminine psychology from the Psyche-Dionysus relation, and the long section on the myth of Psyche in his essay on the symbolism of the ancient tombs.[7]

On the other hand, a significant contribution to the knowledge of the parts synthesized in the myth as it has come down to us was made by Reitzenstein with his discovery of Psyche as an oriental goddess.[8] In an Egyptian magic papyrus Reitzenstein found the figure of Eros[9] as a boy and living god, bearing the epithets "dweller in the palace of heart's desire and lord of the beautiful couch" and "winged dragon." The goddess Psyche, for her part, "gives the universe movement and animation, and one day when Hermes leads her, she will bring it joy"; her partner is an omniscient dragon-monster.

Reitzenstein's reference to the Gnosticism of Apuleius' day is fruitful, but, as we shall see, it does not take us very far. Reitzenstein points to the Gnostic belief that God in-

[6] *Das Mutterrecht*, Vol. II, p. 585.

[7] *Versuch*, p. 94.

[8] Reitzenstein, "Die Göttin Psyche."

[9] On the name Eros *vs.* Amor or Cupid, see my forenote, above, p. 56. Also see Jahn, *Bericht über einige auf Eros und Psyche bezügliche Kunstwerke*; Pagenstecher, "Eros und Psyche"; and Reitzenstein, "Eros und Psyche in der altägyptisch-griechischen Kleinkunst."

visibly, but quite carnally, consorts with the soul of the elect, who from him receives the seed of immortality. Amid distress and temptation the soul must keep faith with this invisible bridegroom, if it is really to behold God after the death of the flesh and celebrate a heavenly marriage with Him.[10] Reitzenstein aptly quotes Philo[11] as saying that "in the mystery of Bacchus that state of ecstasy is designated as a being-violated by Eros," and points to certain modern folk beliefs, such as the Egyptian notion of a *zar*, or spirit, to whom a maiden must actually be given in marriage. The states of "possession" by a spirit, known to us from the demonology of all times,[12] may be considered in the same context.

But this means that we have to do with an archetypal process which is enacted between the feminine and an invisible masculine spirit, a process which operates in all mystical experience, and can of course be found in all the "sources."

On closer scrutiny the similarity of these "sources" to the myth of Psyche is almost overshadowed by an equal or greater divergency; and, though we cannot stop to demonstrate it here, we find that the similarity is for the most part archetypal, while the divergence is specific. This is true, for example, of the relation between our myth and Reitzenstein's Gnostic myth, in which Psyche is abducted by the prince of darkness but finally redeemed by the pleromatic supreme godhead.

---

[10] Reitzenstein, "Die Göttin Psyche," p. 25.

[11] *De vita contemplativa*, 473 M.

[12] Cf. Ansky's interesting play *The Dybbuk, or Between Two Worlds*, which is based on such a "possession" of love.

The archetypal dualism of Iranian Gnosticism is something entirely different from the twofold structure of Eros in our myth, where the essential is precisely the opposite, namely a synthesis of opposites as experienced in the partner, in Eros. We might say very much the same in regard to Reitzenstein's construction of an oriental myth of Psyche, according to which Psyche has slain Eros and undertakes her journey to the underworld in order to bring him the water of life. To begin with, this oriental mythologem, known to us from Ishtar and Tammuz, has nothing to do with the myth of Psyche,[13] since the accents are exactly reversed. Even if an oriental mythologem of this sort had influenced the tale of Psyche, it would—and this is the crucial point—have been elaborated in an entirely different way. The same applies to Kerényi's attempt to relate "the goddess with the bowl"[14] to Psyche. If he is right in setting up a parallel between the "goddess with the bowl" on the one hand and Ariadne and Theseus-Dionysus on the other, and interpreting the bowl as that which "requires fulfillment" by the masculine, this attitude of receiving and waiting for redemption forms a direct antithesis to what is the very crux of the Psyche myth, namely the *activity* of Psyche, who creates her own redemption. As we have shown, this "need for fulfillment" can apply only to the final situation. But this mystical situation is itself archetypal, and has no need of a comparatist "derivation."

[13] The Egyptian terra cotta of Psyche and Eros which Reitzenstein ("Die Göttin Psyche") and after him Kerényi ("Die Göttin mit der Schale") interpret as representing Psyche slaying Eros shows nothing of the sort.

[14] "Die Göttin mit der Schale."

Thus only the vaguest connection can be found between the oriental mythologem and our myth of Psyche. The ancient Greek folk tale of Psyche presents a far closer parallel. Although we have no text of this tale, we know for certain from its numerous reflections in ancient art that in it Eros not only brings suffering to Psyche, often shown as a moth (for this is the meaning of the word *psyche*), but that he himself is tormented by Psyche in exactly the same way.[15] This shows the antiquity of certain central motifs of our Psyche myth, which are not to be found in the above-mentioned oriental myths. The idea that the human soul is not passively cleansed and purified, but actively imposes the same purification upon the loving Eros, is prefigured in the folk tale and achieves its full meaning in the myth of Psyche. Here it is not Psyche alone who is transformed; her destiny is indissolubly intertwined with that of Eros, her partner. We have then a myth of the relation between man and woman.

To follow the mythological history of this Eros is far beyond our scope. But it is no accident that his myth should always be connected with "matriarchal mysteries." Eros as son of Aphrodite has been compared to Horus,[16] and this parallel shows his connection with the great sphere of the matriarchal mysteries, dominated by Isis, mother of Horus. Furthermore, recent scholars believe[17] the ancient Greek Eros to have been a successor of the young pre-Hellenic Cretan god, corresponding to such divine youths as Adonis and Attis, with their evi-

[15] Jahn, *Bericht.*
[16] Persson, *The Religion of Greece in Prehistoric Times*, p. 119.
[17] Ibid., p. 151.

dent relation to the Great Mother. This Cretan origin of Eros takes us back to the prepatriarchal, that is, matriarchal stratum of the Mediterranean cultures, whose beginnings go back to prehistoric times.[18]

In this connection there remains one vitally important parallel: the Eros introduced in Plato's *Symposium* by Diotima, whom Socrates plainly characterizes as a priestess of feminine mysteries.[19] In his study on the "Great Daemon of the Symposium,"[20] Kerényi has brilliantly interpreted this Eros and his mystery. The work of the mystery is "to engender and bear in the beautiful," to bear "a mysterious child who impregnates the body as well as the soul by his presence," and this pregnancy bears witness to the presence and activity of Eros. The fulfillment of this pregnancy, the end of Eros' pain, is "birth in beauty." The highest form of this birth, as Socrates learns from the matriarchal mysteries of Diotima, is self-birth in the "rebirth of the initiate as a divine being."

There is no doubt that if Apuleius, as a Platonist, understood Diotima's mystery of Eros in the sense set forth by Kerényi, he must have related it to the mysteries of Isis, the Eleusinian mysteries, and the ancient folk tale about the suffering Psyche. Gnostic and oriental influences may also have played their part. And yet, at every step in this mythical tale, we are overwhelmed by

[18] Levy, *The Gate of Horn*; Thomson, *The Prehistoric Aegean*.
[19] It is again to Bachofen that we owe our knowledge of the connection between the Mantinean Diotima and the Pelasgian-matriarchal, that is, pre-Hellenic, cultural sphere. (Bachofen, *Das Mutterrecht*, Vol. II, pp. 844 ff.)
[20] *Der grosse Daimon des Symposion.*

its unity and the unity of the feminine psychology which flows from it, and which cannot have been derived entirely from source material alone. It becomes understandable only against the background of an archaic "matriarchal psychology," an operative psychic stratum discernible in any number of myths, rites, and mysteries.[21]

And now perhaps we are in a position to understand how a man should have been able to produce the tale of Psyche, this central document of feminine psychology, for there is no doubt that he did not merely transmit it, but also helped to give it form. Seen objectively, various streams of archaic matriarchal psychology have converged in it. Through the mystery of Isis, Egypt exerted a strong influence on the Hellenistic mysteries of initiation; while the Eleusinian mysteries, as well as the Greek and pre-Hellenic mysteries of Eros, stem from the matriarchal, pre-Hellenic Mediterranean culture, and influenced Plato and the Platonist Apuleius through Mantinea-Diotima. Similarly, the myths and mysteries of Aphrodite are not Greek but come from the Near Eastern precinct of the Great Mother, of whom all the Greek goddesses represent partial aspects. The oriental mythologems of the Great Mother and her young son, (that of Ishtar, for example) are likewise matriarchal, and the Gnostic myths, with their archetypal spirit-heaven world, clearly reveal the struggle of a rising masculine patriarchal ideology against the domination of the archetype of the Great Mother.[22]

For Apuleius, as for many men of his time, this ob-

[21] See my *The Great Mother*, pp. 281 ff.
[22] My *Origins*, pp. 163 f., 460 f., etc.

jective cultural datum became subjective experience through his initiation into the mysteries of Isis, which he describes in his *Golden Ass*, and in which matriarchal psychology becomes masculine experience. But another reason why with Apuleius the experience of religious initiation became the personal experience of the man is that he was one of those creative men who, like the feminine, must give birth, one of those "whom Psyche guides."

LIST OF WORKS CITED

LIST OF WORKS CITED

AELIAN [Claudius Aelianus]. *Varia historia*. In: *Works*, Vol. II. Edited by Rudolf Hercher. Leipzig, 1866.

ANSKY, S., pseud. [Solomon Rappoport]. *The Dybbuk, or Between Two Worlds*. Translated from the Yiddish by Henry G. Alsberg and Winifred Katzin. New York, 1926.

BACHOFEN, JOHANN JAKOB. *Das Mutterrecht*. (Gesammelte Werke, Vols. II and III.) Basel, 1948. 2 vols.

——. *Versuch über die Gräbersymbolik der Alten*. (Gesammelte Werke, Vol. IV.) Basel, 1954.

BRIFFAULT, ROBERT. *The Mothers*. London and New York, 1927. 3 vols.

DEUSSEN, PAUL (tr.). *Sechzig Upanishad's des Veda*. Leipzig, 1897.

DIBELIUS, MARTIN. "Die Isisweihe bei Apuleius und verwandte Initiations-Riten." *Sitzungsberichte der Heidelberger Akademie der Wissenschaften*, 1917, no. 4.

EVANS-WENTZ, W. Y. (ed.). *The Tibetan Book of the Dead*. Lama Kazi Dawa-Samdup's English rendering. 2nd edition, London, 1949.

FRIEDLÄNDER, LUDWIG. *Darstellungen aus der Sittengeschichte Roms in der Zeit von August bis zum Ausgang der Antonine*. Leipzig, 1910. 4 vols.

GRAVES, ROBERT (tr.). *The Transformations of Lucius, otherwise known as The Golden Ass, by Lucius Apuleius*. London and New York, 1950.

ILMER, FLORENS (ed.). *Einleitung zu Apuleius, der Goldene Esel*. Berlin, 1920.

JAHN, OTTO. *Bericht über einige auf Eros und Psyche bezügliche Kunstwerke*. 1851.

JUNG, C. G. *Psychology and Alchemy*. Translated by R. F. C. Hull. (Collected Works, Vol. 12.) New York and London, 1953.

——. "The Psychology of the Child Archetype." In: JUNG

and KERÉNYI, C., *Essays on a Science of Mythology*, q.v.

——. "The Relations between the Ego and the Unconscious." In: *Two Essays on Analytical Psychology.* (Collected Works, Vol. 7.) New York and London, 1953.

—— and KERÉNYI, C. *Essays on a Science of Mythology.* Translated by R. F. C. Hull. New York and London, 1950/1951. [London edn. titled *Introduction to a Science of Mythology.*]

—— and WILHELM, RICHARD. *The Secret of the Golden Flower.* Translated by Cary F. Baynes. New York and London, 1931.

KERÉNYI, C. "Die Göttin mit der Schale." In: *Niobe.* Zurich, 1949.

——. *Der grosse Daimon des Symposion.* (Albae Vigiliae, XIII. Amsterdam, 1942.

——. "The Psychological Aspects of the Kore." In: JUNG, C. G. and KERÉNYI, C. *Essays on a Science of Mythology*, q.v.

——. *Töchter der Sonne.* Zurich, 1944.

——. "Urmensch und Mysterien." *Eranos-Jahrbuch 1947* (Zurich, 1948).

LEVY, G. RACHEL. *The Gate of Horn.* Chicago and London, 1948.

LÉVY-BRUHL, LUCIEN. *Primitive Mentality.* Translated by Lilian A. Clare. London and New York, 1923.

NEUMANN, ERICH. "Die Bedeutung des Erdarchetyps für die Neuzeit." *Eranos-Jahrbuch 1954* (Zurich, 1955).

——. *The Great Mother.* Translated by Ralph Manheim. New York and London, 1955.

——. "Die mythische Welt und der Einzelne." *Eranos-Jahrbuch 1949* (Zurich, 1950). Also in: *Kulturentwicklung und Religion.* (Umkreisung der Mitte, Vol. I.) Zurich, 1953.

——. *The Origins and History of Consciousness.* Translated by R. F. C. Hull. New York and London, 1954.

——. "Die psychologischen Stadien der weiblichen Entwicklung." In: *Zur Psychologie des Weiblichen*, q.v.

——. "Über den Mond und das matriarchale Bewusstsein." *Eranos-Jahrbuch*, Sonderband, Vol. XVIII (Zurich, 1950). Also in: *Zur Psychologie des Weiblichen*, q.v.

——. *Zur Psychologie des Weiblichen*. (Umkreisung der Mitte, Vol. II.) Zurich, 1953.

PAGENSTECHER, RUDOLF. "Eros und Psyche." *Sitzungsberichte der Heidelberger Akademie der Wissenschaften*, 1911, no. 9.

PERSSON, A. W. *The Religion of Greece in Prehistoric Times*. (Sather Classical Lectures, No. 17.) Berkeley and Los Angeles, 1942.

PHILIPPSON, PAULA. *Thessalische Mythologie*. Zurich, 1944.

PHILO JUDAEUS. *De vita contemplativa*. Translated by F. H. Colson in the Loeb Classical Library *Philo*, Vol. IX. Cambridge, Mass., 1941.

PICARD, CHARLES. "Die Ephesia von Anatolien." *Eranos-Jahrbuch 1938* (Zurich, 1939).

REITZENSTEIN, RICHARD. "Eros und Psyche in der altägyptisch-griechischen Kleinkunst." *Sitzungsberichte der Heidelberger Akademie der Wissenschaften*, 1914, no. 12.

——. "Die Göttin Psyche in der hellenistischen und frühchristlichen Literatur." *Sitzungsberichte der Heidelberger Akademie der Wissenschaften*, 1917, no. 10.

——. *Das Märchen von Amor und Psyche bei Apuleius*. Berlin and Leipzig, 1912.

RILKE, RAINER MARIA. *Poems*. Translated from the German by J. B. Leishman. London, 1934.

ROHDE, ERWIN. *Der griechische Roman und seine Vorläufer*. 3rd edn., Leipzig, 1914.

ROSE, HERBERT J. *A Handbook of Greek Mythology*. 5th edn., London, 1953.

THOMSON, GEORGE. *The Prehistoric Aegean*. (Studies in Ancient Greek Society, Vol. I.) London, 1949.

UNGNAD, ARTHUR. *Die Religion der Babylonier und Assyrier.* Jena, 1921.

WEINREICH, OTTO. "Das Märchen von Amor und Psyche." In: FRIEDLÄNDER, q.v., Vol. IV, sec. 10.

WILHELM, RICHARD. See JUNG, C. G., and WILHELM, RICHARD.

INDEX

INDEX

Page references in italic are to Apuleius' tale; the others are to the Commentary.

A

abduction, 63
Achaea, *47*
Admetus, 65–68
Adonis, 61, 158
Aelian, 99*n*
aggression, 63, 81, 100
Alcestis, 65–68
alchemy, 144–45
Alexandrine Aphrodite, 62
Amazons, 79, 82*n*, 99
America, 112
Amor, see Eros
anima, 83, 101*n*, 141–42&*n*, 151*n*
animals, 63, 77, 78, 87, 90, 95, 96*n*, 108, 111, 112, 135; *see also* ants; ass; birds; bull; Cerberus; dog; dolphin; doves; dragon; eagle; goat; hawk; insects; moth; rams; sea mew; serpent; whale; wolves
animus, 134–35, 140
anointing, 84
Ansky, S. (Solomon Rappoport), 156*n*
Anteros, 80*n*
ants, *42*, 95, 115, 126
Aphrodite (=Venus in tale), *3, 26, 52, 53,* 80&*n*, 85, 86, 138, 139, 142, 143, 147, 160; Alexandrine, 62; aspects of, 116–17, 122–24, 126–28, 136; birth of, *3,* 58–59, 90; jealousy of, *4–5, 8, 57,* 58–61, 86–93; labors imposed on Psyche, *see* labors of Psyche; as self, 127–28, 130,

136; vengeance of, *5, 27, 31–41, 57,* 60–61, 69
Apollo, *53;* oracle of, *6–7, 22, 57, 61, 74,* 115, 134
Arabian Nights, 70, 114
archetypes: Aphrodite and Persephone as, 116–17, 122–24, 126–28, 136; and engulfment, 74*n;* father (Zeus), 142; and Gnosticism, 156–57; Great Mother, 87*ff,* 127–31; marriage of death, *see* death, marriage of; and mysteries, 138–39; and Psyche, 141–45; relation of man and woman, 108–110, 113; splitting of, 129; world of, 86; *see also* symbols
Argos, *37*
Ariadne, 157
Aristophontes, 153*n*
arrow, *5, 26, 27, 32ff, 51, 77ff, 83, 84*
Artemis of Ephesus, 82*n*
ass, *47, 49,* 87, 150
assumption of Mary, 144
Attis, 158
Aucnus, 114*n*
Aurora, *43*
autochthony, 95

B

Babylonia, 87, 116
Bacchus, mystery of, 156
Bachofen, J. J., 86&*n,* 95&*n,* 108, 114*n,* 147–48, 154–55, 159*n*
Bad Father, 128
Bad Mother, 92, 93, 118, 128–30

HARPER TORCHBOOKS / The University Library

HARPER TORCHBOOKS / The Academy Library

HARPER TORCHBOOKS / The Bollingen Library

HARPER TORCHBOOKS / The Cloister Library

HARPER TORCHBOOKS / The Science Library